A CONCISE GUIDE TO

Intraoperative Monitoring

A CONCISE GUIDE TO

Intraoperative Monitoring

GEORGE ZOURIDAKIS, PH.D.
DEPARTMENT OF NEUROSURGERY
UNIVERSITY OF TEXAS-HOUSTON MEDICAL SCHOOL

ANDREW C. PAPANICOLAOU, PH.D.
DEPARTMENT OF NEUROSURGERY
UNIVERSITY OF TEXAS-HOUSTON MEDICAL SCHOOL

CRC Press
Boca Raton   London   New York   Washington, D.C.

Library of Congress Cataloging-in-Publication Data

Zouridakis, George
    A concise guide to intraoperative monitoring/ George Zouridakis, Andrew C. Papanicolaou.
        p. ; cm.
    Includes bibliographical references and index.
    ISBN 0-8493-0886-0 (alk. paper)
    1. Biomedical engineering. 2. Intraoperative monitoring. 3. Electrophysiology. 4.
Neurophysiology. I. Papanicolaou, Andrew C. II. Title.
    [DNLM: 1. Monitoring, Intraoperative—methods. 2. Electrophysiology. WO 181 Z91c 2000]
R856. .Z68 2000
617'.91—dc21   00-046750

Visit the CRC Press Web site at www.crcpress.com

Preface

Intraoperative electrophysiological recordings are gradually becoming part of standard medical practice, mainly because they offer an objective and effective way to assess the functional integrity of the nervous system of patients during the course of orthopedic, neurological, or vascular surgery. Continuous monitoring of bioelectrical activity not only can avert damage of neurological structures that are at risk during certain surgical maneuvers, but also allows identification of specific neuronal structures and landmarks that cannot be easily recognized on anatomical grounds only.

Early applications of intraoperative monitoring were limited to a neuroprotective role. Today, however, monitoring not only decreases the risk for permanent neurological deficits but also provides surgeons with continuous information pertaining to the functional integrity of neuronal structures at risk and allows them to modify their actions accordingly in an effort to achieve optimal results.

Intraoperative monitoring is still not perfect. In fact, results are affected by several factors that may lead to false positive and negative judgments or interpretations. However, until more advanced procedures become available and practical, monitoring will remain a very useful and clinically valid procedure that can improve surgical outcome.

This book, based on our experience with the intraoperative monitoring service at Hermann Hospital and on that of others, introduces the various recording techniques available today, the rationale for their intraoperative use, the basic principles on which they are based, as well as problems typically encountered with their implementation. Specific features of the recorded signals, proper parameter settings for acquisition, and factors that affect the recordings, with emphasis on anesthetic agents and various neuroprotective induced conditions, such as hypothermia and hypotension, are reviewed in detail. Recommendations for procedure implementation, proper interpretation of the recordings, and successful equipment troubleshooting are also given. Finally, each chapter concludes with a series of questions to help the reader review the major points presented in the chapter.

About the Authors

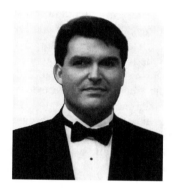

George Zouridakis, Ph.D., is Associate Professor and Director of the Bioimaging Laboratory in the Department of Neurosurgery of the University of Texas-Houston Medical School. He has served as a founding member of the Intraoperative Monitoring Service at Memorial-Hermann Hospital. Dr. Zouridakis's clinical activities currently focus on functional neurosurgery and brain mapping. His research interests involve the development of techniques for image processing, pattern recognition, automated detection, and modeling of biosignals using nonlinear dynamical analysis and fuzzy decision making. In the area of medical imaging, Dr. Zouridakis has developed a graduate course that he currently teaches at Rice University. Since the early stages of his career, he has received several awards and he is also listed in *Who's Who in America.*

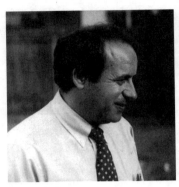

A.C. Papanicolaou, Ph.D., is a member of the American Society of Neurophysiological Monitoring and Professor and Director of the Division of Clinical Neurosciences in the Neurosurgery Department of the University of Texas-Houston Medical School and the Magnetoencephalography Center at the Memorial-Hermann Hospital. During the past 20 years Dr. Papanicolaou has worked and published extensively in the areas of brain electrophysiology, neuropsychology, cognitive neurosciences and functional brain imaging, the fundamentals of which he has presented in a recent textbook. In 1993, he organized and directed the Intraoperative Monitoring Service at Memorial-Hermann Hospital where he still contributes as a member of the pallidotomy team.

Contents

chapter 1

Introduction

1.1 Intraoperative Monitoring

Electrophysiological recordings during orthopedic, neurological, and vascular surgery are gradually becoming part of standard medical practice, mainly because these procedures, unlike other intraoperative techniques such as X-ray and ultrasound imaging which provide information on the anatomical status of a structure, provide information regarding the *functional integrity* of the nervous system of a patient who, typically, is anesthetized and therefore cannot be neurologically examined. The value of these procedures, which are collectively known as *intraoperative monitoring* (IOM), stems from the fact that they are *practical* (no active patient participation is required), *reliable* (normal recordings are known to be very stable over time), and *sensitive* (they can promptly detect small changes in the activity of the nervous system).

Typical recordings include monitoring of the spontaneous electrical activity of the brain, which is recorded on the scalp as the electroencephalogram (EEG), and that of muscles, which can be obtained by placing electrodes in the vicinity of contracting muscles and is referred to as an electromyogram (EMG). However, the most commonly recorded signals in the operating room are *evoked potentials* (EPs), which are the electrophysiological responses of the nervous system to external stimulation.

Early applications of intraoperative monitoring were limited to only a few tests. The original use of somatosensory EPs in the late 1970s was to monitor spinal cord function during Harrington rod instrumentation for scoliosis [16, 51]. At that time, attempts to preserve facial nerve function led to monitoring facial muscle contractions through recordings of EMG activity [14]. Later, after their discovery in humans [27], auditory brainstem responses (ABRs) were among the modalities routinely monitored during surgical operations for acoustic tumors [13, 22] with the intention to preserve hearing and vestibular nerve functions. Currently, additional tests have been developed specifically for intraoperative use, covering a wider range of applications.

1.2   Use

In general, the application of these procedures intraoperatively serves a dual purpose. The first purpose, already mentioned earlier, is to avert damage of neuronal structures that are at risk during certain surgical maneuvers. For instance, as will be described in greater detail in Chapter 8, during surgery for scoliosis (see Section 8.2), monitoring of the spinal cord through EPs can provide early warnings of impending damage due to misplaced instrumentation or to unintended manipulation of the cord, like for example, excessive distraction. Or, during a carotid endarterectomy (see Section 9.5), potentially dangerous decreases in cortical blood perfusion rates can be inferred from EEG and EP recordings and corrected in time.

The second purpose is to identify specific neuronal structures and landmarks that cannot be easily recognized on anatomical grounds only. For example, during surgery for epilepsy, identification of the *central sulcus* which separates the motor and sensory areas of the cerebral cortex can be achieved by delineating the somatosensory area using a simple EP test (see Section 9.7).

1.3   Rationale

Events occurring in the external environment, such as sounds and lights, are detected by the sense organs and information about them is transmitted to the brain in the form of electrical signals through various sensory neural pathways. The arrival of these signals in the brain gives rise to certain patterns of brain activity, provided that these pathways are structurally and functionally intact. Consequently, examination of these patterns of brain activity can provide valuable information regarding the integrity of the neural structures that constitute the pathway.

In general, two consequences of surgical intervention, however infrequent, can compromise the functional integrity of the nervous system and possibly lead to post-operative neurological deficits: *ischemia* and *mechanical injury*. These insults are typically manifested as a change in the morphology, amplitude, or frequency content of the electrophysiological signals being recorded. Continuous measurement of these waveform parameters and comparison with pre-established normative values allows one to assess, on-line, the functional integrity of neuronal structures over time.

Therefore, intraoperative neurophysiological monitoring provides an objective way to *detect* and *quantify*, instant by instant, changes in the functional status of neuro-logical structures early enough, so that actions can be taken to possibly reverse the effects of ischemia, prevent permanent mechanical injury, and restore normal func-tion. And since the information is provided in real time, through monitoring one can also assess the efficacy of a corrective action, e.g., removal of an arterial clamp that had previously resulted in local ischemia (see Figure 9.18). Monitoring can also help the surgeon to assess the effectiveness of surgical intervention, such as, for example, the adequacy of root decompression in the case of a radiculopathy (see Section 8.3).

1.4 Types of Tests

Intraoperative monitoring employs recordings of two main categories of bioelectric signals: spontaneous activity and evoked responses. Examples of the former category are the spontaneous activity of the brain (EEG) (see Section 6.2) and of muscles (EMG) (see Section 6.3). Recordings in the latter category are obtained through external stimulation of a neural pathway. Typical stimuli used in sensory stimulation consist of small electrical shocks, clicking sounds, and flashes of light, which result in the familiar somatosensory, auditory, and visual evoked potentials, respectively. Similarly, electrical or magnetic stimulation of a motor pathway gives rise to the so-called motor evoked potentials.

Evoked responses usually are very small compared to the ongoing activity, thus averaging of a large number of them is necessary to obtain clear response waveforms. Somatosensory and auditory evoked potentials are examples of averaged responses. In certain cases, however, individual stimuli result in large responses, therefore, averaging is not necessary. This is the case, for example, of an electrical stimulus delivered to spinal nerves resulting in high-amplitude responses known as triggered EMG (see Section 7.8).

Depending on the site of stimulation, evoked responses can be recorded from the brain, the spinal cord, a peripheral nerve, or a muscle. Unfortunately, there is no single monitoring procedure that can be used in all circumstances. The type of test to be used and the sites of recording and stimulation are chosen on a case by case basis, depending on what structures are at risk in the context of a particular surgical procedure. And, very often, it is necessary to employ multiple tests simultaneously, in order to maximize the sensitivity of IOM.

1.5 Affecting Factors

In addition to surgical manipulation which, unintentionally, may result in ischemia or mechanical injury, neurophysiological recordings are also affected by other *perisurgical* factors, such as blood pressure, body temperature and, most importantly, the anesthesia regime. Of course, there is always the additional possibility of a technical problem which may result in a drastic change in the recordings. Familiarity with all these factors is necessary for proper interpretation of any activity changes that might be detected during the course of surgery.

Most anesthetic drugs influence neurophysiological signals because of the effects they have on cerebral blood flow, perfusion, and metabolic rate. Hence, collaboration of the monitoring team with the anesthesiologist is critical in developing a proper anesthesia plan suitable for both the surgical *and* the monitoring procedures. An overview of anesthesia management during neurological, orthopedic, and vascular surgery will be given in Section 5.2.

1.6   Interpretation

Besides the above-mentioned factors that affect neurophysiological recordings, there are additional ones related to artifacts. Extraneous biological noise, such as the electrocardiographic (ECG) or muscle activity, electrical interference, like the omnipresent 60 Hz activity, or equipment failure, for instance a faulty stimulating device, will all contribute to the difficulty in correctly interpreting the recordings and the ability of differentiating artifacts from changes due to ischemia or mechanical injury.

In general, ischemia and mechanical insult will result in (1) a decrease in the number of neurons responding to stimulation, and (2) desynchronization of neuronal firing. From an electrophysiological point of view, these changes are detected as a reduction in the amplitude, an increase in the latency, and an overall change in the morphology of a waveform. Although there are no exact values of amplitude and possibly latency changes that absolutely predict neurologic outcome [6], for each test there are recommended values which can be used as a "rule of thumb" for warning the surgical team about a significant change in the recordings.

As will be explained in later chapters, careful observation of the context in which signal changes occur, including surgical maneuvers (tissue retraction, instrumentation placement, etc.) and other perisurgical factors (bolus injection of drugs, decreased blood pressure, etc.), as well as communication with the surgeon and the anesthesiologist, allows one to correctly assess the importance of these changes.

1.7   Usefulness

The merits of intraoperative monitoring have been extensively reported in the literature from different institutions worldwide and for a variety of types of surgery.

For example, several studies have shown the benefits of spinal cord monitoring during surgery for scoliosis [32, 53, 57, 60, 68]. A large multicenter survey found that such monitoring has a *sensitivity* (the true positive out of the total true positive and false negative change detections) of 92% and a *specificity* (the true negative out of the total true negative and false positive change detections) of 98.9%, with an even higher negative predictive value of 99.93% (the true negative out of true negative and false negative change detections), indicating that the test is highly likely to be accurate when no changes are detected [53]. Also, in neurovascular cases EP findings were found to be consistent with the clinical outcome [52] and could be used intraoperatively for early detection of ischemia and for assessing the efficacy of surgical countermeasures [40], thus allowing for overall safer operations [61].

Similarly, intraoperative monitoring of compound nerve action potentials from various cranial nerves has proven to be an invaluable tool in avoiding neurological damage and preserving function of the facial, cochlear, trigeminal, spinal accessory, and oculomotor nerves [30, 47, 62, 75].

Also, auditory brainstem responses (ABRs) have found widespread clinical applications in assessing the integrity of the peripheral auditory structures and brainstem pathways [38] and have made brain retraction, which is required for adequate exposure during many intracranial procedures, a much less common source of morbidity [4].

However, beyond the main objective of early detection of possible neurological complications to allow for their timely correction, intraoperative monitoring has other advantages. Continuous feedback regarding neurological function provides the medical team with additional reassurance and allows the surgeons to carry out the operation in an optimal way [47] attempting, for instance, more aggressive maneuvers that otherwise they would not risk attempting [53]. Also, certain high-risk patients previously regarded as inoperable can now be considered as candidates for surgery.

1.8   Cost Effectiveness

It would seem obvious that if intraoperative monitoring can decrease the risk of permanent postoperative neurological deficit, or the time it takes to perform an operation, then the cost related to the service would be justified. In economic terms, however, even when the cost of suffering is not included, it has been estimated that the use of intraoperative monitoring in certain cases is clinically cost-effective as the risk of postoperative complications approaches 1% [53].

Nevertheless, it is important to keep the surgical cost within reasonable limits, by carefully selecting to perform monitoring in patients who would *likely* benefit from it as opposed to performing it indiscriminately just because it is available.

1.9   Personnel

Guidelines for proper intraoperative monitoring have been set forth by the American Electroencephalographic Society [6] and include recommendations for equipment, personnel, and documentation. Selection of proper personnel to perform intraoperative monitoring is critical. It has been found that experience of the monitoring team is the primary predictor of the rate of neurological deficits. Specifically, teams with the least experience had significantly higher rates of neurological deficits (twice as high) compared to the most experienced teams [53] .

Typically, one person (a clinical neurophysiologist) is responsible for several operating rooms, while a technologist is available in each room to place electrodes, setup equipment, and monitor the case during the less critical phases of an operation. This is similar to how anesthesia teams are organized in most institutions.

All personnel involved with monitoring should be able to interpret the recordings and communicate the findings to the surgeons. Given that the degree of familiarity of the surgeons with neurophysiological tests varies, communication should be in a way that the surgeons find useful for their purposes. This implies that at least the person responsible for monitoring, in addition to being able to troubleshoot and solve problems with equipment, should have a strong background in clinical neurophysiology and anatomy, as well as, knowledge about the specific surgical operation being performed.

1.10   Equipment

The choice of equipment for intraoperative monitoring is very important. A typical system consists of a portable, self-contained, computer-controlled unit that includes all the components and has the capacity to perform all the operations essential to the task: recording, stimulation, display, signal processing, and data storage.

The equipment should have several desirable features which, although not absolutely necessary for routine clinical recordings, are of special importance for intraoperative recordings. For instance, it should allow for simultaneous multimodality recordings, such as auditory and somatosensory evoked responses, to meet the needs of specific operations. However, it should also be easy to use, flexible, and should allow modifications in the recording protocol and display parameters, if necessary, thus permitting fast interpretation of the results.

1.11   Organization of the Book

This book provides an overview of the techniques available for intraoperative use and their application to specific surgical procedures. Chapter 2 provides an introduction to the origin of the electrophysiological signals recorded, and a description of their basic features. Chapter 3 gives a brief review on basic concepts in electricity and the technical characteristics of the recording equipment, while Chapter 4 summarizes the characteristics of the recorded signals and the processing they undergo before they can be interpreted. A short description of the most commonly used anesthetic agents and their effects on electrophysiological signals is given in Chapter 5. Chapter 6 and Chapter 7 describe the most typical tests employed during intraoperative monitoring, and give specific examples of recorded activity. Chapter 8 and Chapter 9 summarize the most common types of spinal and cranial surgery, respectively, as well as the tests to employ for appropriate IOM of the structures at risks. Chapter 10 is dedicated to equipment troubleshooting and the development of intervention strategies. Chapter 11 concludes the book with some final remarks on the usefulness, clinical validity, and cost-effectiveness of IOM.

1.12   Review Questions

1. Define intraoperative monitoring (IOM).

2. What are the most common types of electrophysiological signals recorded intraoperatively?

3. What is the purpose of IOM?

4. On what principles is IOM based?

5. Name the two primary risks to the nervous system associated with surgery.

6. What kind of changes are observed in physiological recordings after an ischemic attack of, or mechanical insult to, neuronal structures?

7. Name the various body structures from which evoked responses can be recorded.

8. What are the factors affecting neurophysiological recordings?

9. What kind of noise affects neurophysiological recordings?

10. What kind of benefits does IOM offer?

11. What is the approximate percentage of postoperative complications in spine surgery?

12. Does experience of the IOM personnel affect the rate of postoperative neurological deficits?

13. What is the most common structure of an IOM team?

14. What responsibilities/abilities should personnel involved with IOM have?

15. Name the main parts of an IOM recording system.

chapter 2

Neurophysiological Background

2.1   Introduction

The science of *anatomy* aims at understanding the architecture of the body as a whole and the structure of its various parts. *Physiology,* on the other hand, is concerned with understanding the mechanisms by which the body performs its various functions. A few common terms used to describe the structure and relative position of all human body parts are introduced in the next section.

During surgery, several neuronal structures are at risk for permanent damage due to surgical manipulation, but continuous recordings of neurophysiological signals provide a reliable and effective way to protect the structural and functional integrity of these structures.

Neurophysiological signals can be divided into two main categories: *spontaneous activity,* such as the EEG and EMG, and *evoked responses.* The latter category includes the familiar evoked potentials (EPs) which are obtained from external stimulation of a sensory neural pathway.

To better understand the nature of the neurophysiological activity and the clinical validity of intraoperative monitoring, the basic mechanisms that give rise to the signals recorded are briefly summarized.

2.2   Organization of the Human Body

2.2.1   Anatomic References

The general form of the human body is bilaterally symmetric, or the two sides are the mirror image of each other. Several common terms used to describe anatomic positions and structures in the body, as well as the relative location of various parts, are summarized in Table 2.1. Most of these terms are self-explanatory. It is worth noticing, however, that the terms "anterior" and "ventral" are synonymous with respect to the spinal cord, but in the brain, *anterior* refers to structures toward the frontal lobes, while *ventral* refers to structures toward the spinal cord (the lower surface of the brain). Similarly, "posterior" and "dorsal" are synonymous with respect to the spinal cord, but in the brain, *posterior* refers to structures toward the occipital lobes, while *dorsal* refers to structures toward the upper surface of the brain.

Table 2.1   Description of
Common Anatomic References

Anterior	In the front part
Posterior	In the back part
Ventral	Toward the belly
Dorsal	Toward the back
Cranial	Toward the head
Caudal	Toward the tail
Medial	Toward the midline
Lateral	Away from the midline
Proximal	Near the reference
Distal	Away from the reference

There are also three planes of reference or sections through the body, which are orthogonal to each other, namely *coronal, sagittal,* and *axial,* that divide the body into front and back, left and right, and upper and lower parts, respectively. The *midsagittal* plane is vertical at the midline, while a closeby parallel plane is often called *parasagittal.* Table 2.2 gives a summary description of the various sections, while Figure 2.1 shows a graphical illustration of the planes through the human brain.

Table 2.2   Description of Common Reference Planes

Coronal, Frontal	Longitudinal plane that divides a structure into front and back parts.
Sagittal	Vertical plane that divides a structure into left and right parts. The midsagittal plane is vertical at the midline.
Axial, Transverse	Horizontal plane that divides a structure into upper and lower parts.

2.2.2   Functional Groups

In spite of great variations in appearance and consistency, the building block of all parts of the human body is the *cell*. Groups of similar cells that perform a specific function form a particular *tissue*. Examples of such formations are the epithelial, connective, muscular, and nervous tissues.

In turn, two or more tissues that are grouped together and perform a highly specialized function form an *organ*. For example, the heart has walls that are composed

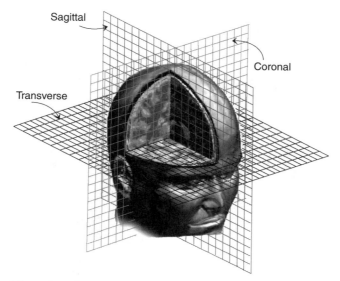

Sagittal

Coronal

Transverse

Figure 2.1   Illustration of the three reference planes.

of muscular and connective tissues, while nervous tissue is distributed through the entire structure.

Furthermore, groups of organs that act together to perform highly complex but specialized functions are known as *systems*. The nervous system is one of many systems found in the human body, and consists of the *brain*, the *spinal cord*, and several peripheral *nerves* and *ganglia*. All these parts are schematically shown in Figure 2.2.

2.3   Origin of Neurophysiological Signals

A cell constitutes not only the *structural* unit but also the *functional* unit of all tissues, organs, and systems. Inside these minute structures take place most of the processes that give rise to activity observed externally.

The *cell membrane*, the boundary around each cell, forms a barrier to molecules that enter or leave the cell through specific structures on it called *channels*. Several chemically active *ions*, that is, molecules carrying an electrical charge, are found in the intracellular and extracellular fluids, the most important of which are sodium (Na^+), potassium (K^+), and chloride (Cl^-). A small patch of cell membrane is schematically shown in Figure 2.3.

A cell's membrane is *selectively permeable*, so that certain ions can cross it through the channels, whereas others cannot. Because of this property, the membrane is *polarized*. That is, the difference in the concentration of positive and negative charges on each side of the membrane results in the so-called *resting membrane potential*, which is approximately 70 μV, with the inside of the cell being negative with respect to the outside, as is schematically shown in the upper right corner of Figure 2.3.

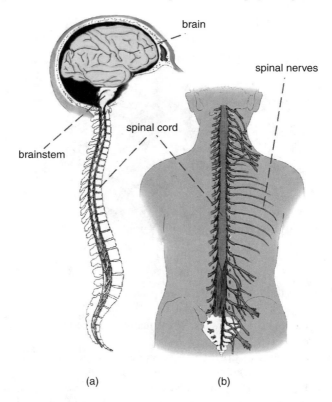

Figure 2.2   The nervous system with the brain, spinal cord, and peripheral nerves; (a) posterior and (b) lateral aspect.

Several events, such as, for example, an external stimulus, can disturb the balance of ion concentration, and this will result in inward and outward movement of ions. For all practical purposes, movement of these ions is equivalent to the flow of electrical current. Indeed, *all* electrophysiological signals are ultimately due to movement of ions across cell membranes. The morphology of the externally recorded signals is primarily determined by the properties of the specific cells and the extracellular fluid surrounding them.

2.4   Spontaneous Activity

2.4.1   Activity of Neural Cells

A *neuron,* shown schematically in Figure 2.4, is the basic structural and functional unit of the nervous system. It is composed of a *cell body,* a very large number of short processes called *dendrites,* and an *axon,* a typically long process that ends in several branches known as axon terminals. Dendrites carry signals toward the cell, whereas

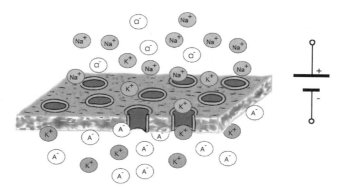

Figure 2.3   A small patch of cell membrane separating the intracellular and extracellular fluid. Several positive and negative ions, such as Na^+, K^+, and Cl^-, cross the membrane through ion channels.

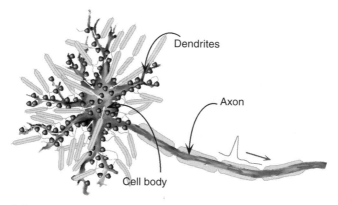

Figure 2.4   Schematic diagram of a cortical neuron.

the axon sends signals away from it. This is schematically shown in Figure 2.4 with yellow and blue arrows, respectively.

When a stimulus is delivered to a neuron, it causes a local change in the permeability of the membrane that results in a net current flow from the outside to the inside of the cell. This, in turn, results in a local change in membrane potential, during which the potential reverses and the inside of the cell becomes positive with respect to the outside. This phenomenon is known as *membrane depolarization*.

Each neuron usually receives signals from several thousand other nerve cells. If the sum of all the signals received exceeds a certain threshold, a much larger depolarization occurs that causes a complete reversal of the voltage across the cell membrane. This then generates an electrical pulse, known as *action potential,* which is self-propagated down the axon of the cell, toward the synaptic end (Figure 2.5).

Transfer of signals from one cell to another is accomplished by a series of electrochemical events at the point of contact between the axonal terminals of the first (or

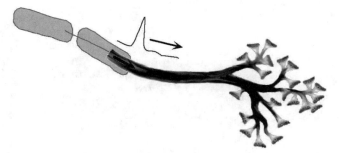

Figure 2.5   Schematic diagram of a cortical neuron's synaptic end.

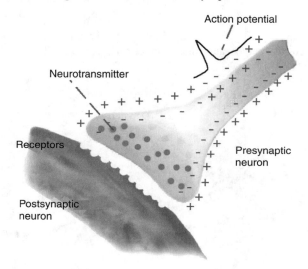

Figure 2.6   Neuronal synapse and generation of a postsynaptic potential.

presynaptic) neuron and the dendrites or the cell body of the second (or *postsynaptic*)
one. This area of contact is called a *synapse,* and is shown schematically in Figure 2.6.

When an action potential reaches the axonal terminals, it causes the release of
a chemical, a *neurotransmitter,* in the synaptic space between adjacent cells. The
neurotransmitter interacts with the next cell and the effect of this interaction is the
generation of a *postsynaptic potential,* which can be either *excitatory* (EPSP) or
inhibitory (IPSP). In the former case, the membrane potential of the second cell is
reduced and brought closer to its firing threshold whereas, in the latter case, it is
increased and brought away from its firing threshold.

In this cell now, if the sum of all the excitatory and inhibitory postsynaptic potentials
exceeds the threshold, then a new action potential will be generated which will travel
down the axon to reach yet another cell. In this fashion, the original pulse may be
propagated down the chain of several cells.

The depolarization of the membrane in the first neuron and the potential reversal
across it are only temporary, since the resting membrane potential and the separation

of ions is rapidly restored by certain cell mechanisms, and the whole process can then be repeated.

2.4.2   *Temporal and Spatial Summation*

An action potential lasts about 2 msec, while a postsynaptic potential is much longer and lasts approximately 25 msec. Thus, it is possible for a postsynaptic neuron to receive a second action potential before the postsynaptic potential generated by the first action potential is over.

Moreover, to initiate an action potential on a postsynaptic neuron, the summation of several EPSPs is required, since the depolarization effect of a single EPSP is small. Summation can be either temporal or spatial. *Temporal* summation occurs when the effects of successive EPSPs generated by the same presynaptic terminal are added together.

Spatial summation, on the other hand, occurs when several presynaptic neurons fire simultaneously, each producing an EPSP at a different place on the postsynaptic neuron, and all these EPSPs are summated.

Every time that the temporal or spatial sum of all postsynaptic potentials exceeds a certain threshold, an action potential is generated.

2.4.3   *Activity of the Cerebral Cortex*

Typically, large numbers of neurons are organized together in functional groups. In the central nervous system, for instance, the outer surface of the brain, the *cerebral cortex,* is composed of an intricate network of neurons that are arranged in layers. A schematic diagram of such an organization is shown in Figure 2.7.

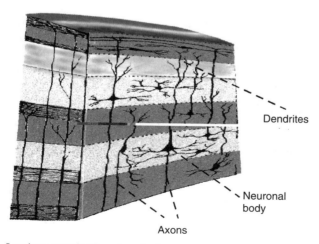

Figure 2.7   Laminar organization of cortical neurons.

The familiar scalp-recorded EEG activity is believed [65] to be due to the processes described in the previous paragraph. It represents the temporal and spatial summation of excitatory and inhibitory postsynaptic potentials generated at the bodies and apical dendrites of *pyramidal cells,* a specific type of neurons found in the cortical network.[1]

2.4.4 *Activity of Peripheral Nerves*

In the peripheral nervous system most of the nerve fibers, or neuronal axons, that travel in the same direction are collected together in bundles, each wrapped in an insulating sheath of *myelin.* In turn, these bundles are "packaged" together with connective tissue to form a *nerve.* Figure 2.8 depicts such a configuration in a peripheral nerve.

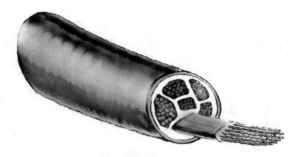

Figure 2.8   A peripheral nerve and its "packaging."

Action potentials traveling along these nerves can be recorded by placing electrodes in their vicinity. For instance, electrical stimulation of the posterior tibial nerve at the ankle (see Section 7.3.6) results in activity (action potentials) which is propagated along the nerve and can be recorded from an electrode placed, for example, at the popliteal fossa or behind the knee.

2.4.5 *Activity of Muscle Cells*

Muscles are composed of large numbers of *muscle fibers* or cells that have the ability to temporarily shorten their length by converting chemical energy into mechanical work. Synchronized contraction of muscle cells produces a movement of some part of the body. The control and coordination of these movements is a major function of the nervous system.

For a skeletal muscle to contract, it must first be stimulated, that is, it must receive an impulse from a motor neuron. A nerve fiber terminating within a muscle branches

---

[1]The cerebral cortex is a highly compact structure with an average thickness of about 2.5 mm and average density of 10^5 cells/mm^2, forming approximately 10^{15} synapses [29].

into many terminal feet, each anchored on the membrane of a muscle fiber. Figure 2.9 shows a peripheral nerve innervating a skeletal muscle. The point of contact between neuron and muscle is analogous to the synapse between nerve cells, and it is known as the *neuromuscular junction.*

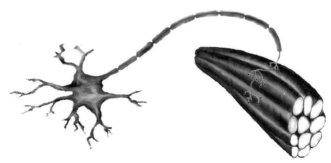

Figure 2.9   A peripheral nerve innervating a skeletal muscle.

Like a nerve cell, the membrane of a muscle fiber is polarized. An impulse arriving at the neuronal end of the neuromuscular junction releases the neurotransmitter *acetylcholine*, which interacts with specialized receptors on the muscle fiber and causes depolarization of its membrane. This depolarization, in turn, triggers a muscle action potential which forces the muscle fiber to contract.

A contracting muscle produces activity that can be recorded with a nearby electrode. A continuous record of this activity is known as *electromyogram* (EMG). If the recorded signals result from direct stimulation of a nerve that innervates the muscle, these signals are also known as *compound muscle action potentials* (CMAPs).

Neutralization of the neurotransmitter released by the motor neuron, or of the receptor on the muscle membrane, prevents the neuronal signals to reach the muscle causing temporary paralysis. The action of *neuromuscular blockers,* drugs that are used intraoperatively during anesthesia, is based on this mechanism. A brief description of these drugs is given in Chapter 5.

2.5   *Evoked Responses*

As mentioned in Chapter 1, evoked responses are obtained from stimulation of a motor or sensory neural pathway. They can be subdivided further into averaged and nonaveraged responses. Averaged responses are typically recorded from the central nervous system, that is the brain and spinal cord, whereas nonaveraged responses are mostly obtained from peripheral structures. Examples of averaged and nonaveraged responses are the well-known somatosensory EPs and the electrically triggered EMG, respectively.

2.5.1 Averaged Responses

Several types of sensory stimulation can elicit EPs, including auditory, visual, and somatosensory. In each modality certain stimulus parameters, such as intensity, duration, and rate, must be properly adjusted to obtain optimal recordings. These issues are discussed in detail in Chapter 7, where exact parameter values specific to each test are also given.

2.5.2 Nonaveraged Responses

Nonaveraged evoked responses can be obtained after direct stimulation, electrical or mechanical, of a motor nerve or a nerve root. These responses are typically recorded as activity from muscles, and they are known as triggered EMG. It is also possible to record nonaveraged responses directly from cranial or peripheral nerves. Details on the procedure, including specific stimulation and recording parameters, are given in Chapter 7.

2.6 Review Questions

1. What are the two major categories of neurophysiological recordings?

2. Briefly explain the meaning of the various anatomic references below:

Anterior		Posterior	
Ventral		Dorsal	
Cranial		Caudal	
Medial		Lateral	
Proximal		Distal	

3. Give the names and describe briefly the three common reference planes.

4. Which are the three most important ions found in the intracellular and extracellular fluids?

5. The membrane of a cell is known to be selectively permeable to ions. What is the overall effect of this property?

6. How are the externally recorded neurophysiological signals generated?

7. Name the basic structural and functional cellular unit found in the nervous system.

8. What happens when a stimulus is delivered locally to a neuron?

9. Describe the phenomenon of membrane depolarization.

10. What is an action potential?

11. What is the name of the point of contact between two neurons?

12. What happens when an action potential reaches the axonal terminals?

13. Is it true that neurotransmitters are always excitatory?

14. What is the name of the outer surface of the brain, and what kind of cells are found in it?

15. How is the scalp-recorded EEG generated?

16. Describe briefly the structure of a nerve.

17. What is the building block of a muscle and what is its characteristic property?

18. What is the relationship between a skeletal muscle and a motor neuron?

19. What is the name of the neurotransmitter released at the neuromuscular junction?

20. What is the action of neuromuscular blockers, i.e., of those drugs commonly used during anesthesia that cause temporary paralysis?

21. How are evoked responses produced?

22. Do all evoked responses represent averaged activity?

chapter 3

Instrumentation

3.1 Introduction

Intraoperative monitoring requires specialized equipment capable of recording different types of neurophysiological signals, including EEG, EMG, and evoked responses. A typical system includes one or more programmable devices that can deliver auditory, visual, and electrical stimuli of variable amplitude, duration, and rate; various types of electrodes for delivering electrical stimuli and for recording electrophysiological activity from the scalp, nerves, and muscles; a head box for selecting among different electrode groups to be connected to the amplifiers; a set of amplifiers; a display monitor; a printer; and often a modem or network connection for remote monitoring. All parts are connected to a computer which, depending on the kind of recordings, controls stimulus delivery, data collection, filtering, averaging, display, printing, as well as remote transmission and permanent storage of the data.

Essential to the recording of electrophysiological activity are the characteristics of the recording electrodes and the appropriate setup of the amplifiers. The details are given in the next several sections.

However, to help the reader understand better the relationship between the electrophysiological activity and the signals displayed on the computer screen, a brief introduction on electrical concepts and the characteristics of basic circuits is given first.

3.2 Basic Concepts

3.2.1 Structure of Matter

All matter consists of *atoms*. In turn, atoms are composed of smaller particles, namely *neutrons, protons,* and *electrons*. Neutrons do not carry a charge, whereas protons and electrons carry a positive and a negative charge, respectively, and thus, they determine the electrical properties of matter. Furthermore, protons and neutrons form the *nucleus* in the center of the atom, while electrons revolve about the nucleus in elliptical orbits.

One fundamental law of electricity, *Coulomb's Law*, states that, "like charges repel and unlike charges attract each other" and explains the bond between the nucleus and the orbiting electrons that exists in the atom. The strength of this bond decreases as the distance of an electron from the nucleus increases. Additionally, this strength differs from element to element and ultimately determines whether an element is a *conductor* or an *insulator.*

3.2.2   Electrical Currents

In conductors, electrons in the outer orbits form very weak bonds with the nucleus. Thus, under the influence of an external filed, they can move *almost* freely, and this electron movement constitutes an *electrical current.* However, as electrons move in the conductor, they collide with nuclei and other electrons that are not free. Electrons, therefore, do not move entirely freely, but the conductor itself exerts some opposition to the current flow that is called *resistance.*

Current is measured in units of Amperes (A). In the case of electrophysiological signals, more common units are fractions of the Ampere, namely the *milli*ampere (mA), where $1\ mA = \frac{1\ A}{1,000}$, and the *micro*ampere (μA), where $1\ \mu A = \frac{1\ A}{1,000,000}$.

The unit of measure of resistance is the Ohm (Ω). Some common multiple units are the *kilo*ohm (kΩ), where 1 kΩ = 1,000 Ω, and the *mega*ohm (MΩ), where 1 MΩ = 1,000,000 Ω.

3.2.3   Resistors

The amount of current in a electronic circuit is controlled by inserting certain components called *resistors.* By construction, resistors are composed of a mixture of conducting and nonconducting material, and thus their resistance can be specified exactly.[1]

When a resistor is connected to a voltage generator, such as, for example, a battery, a flow of electrons, or current, is established, due to the so-called *electromotive force* that exists between the battery's poles. This force is also known as *potential difference* or *voltage.* Voltage is measured in units of volts (V), common subdivisions of which are the millivolt (mV) and the microvolt (μV).

3.2.4   Direct and Alternating Currents

Considering current flow, if the voltage generator provides a constant electromotive force causing electrons to move in a single direction, the result is a *direct current* (dc). In a different type of generator, current flows momentarily in one direction, reverses itself, and then flows in the opposite direction. Such a generator gives rise to an *alternating current* (ac). Current reversal is periodic, and typically occurs 60 times per second, resulting in the familiar 60 Hz cycle artifact seen in many neurophysiological recordings (see Section 10.3). The symbols typically used for direct and alternating current generators are shown in Figure 3.1(a) and Figure 3.1(b), respectively.

---

[1]*Resistors,* i.e., the electronic components, present *resistance,* but often the two terms are used interchangeably.

3.2.5   Ohm's Law

Figure 3.1(c) shows a simple circuit in which a resistor is connected to a voltage generator. There are three electrical measurements that can be obtained from the

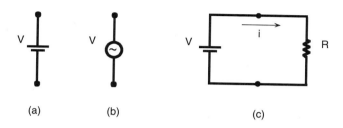

(a)   (b)   (c)

Figure 3.1   Electrical symbol for (a) a direct and (b) an alternating current generator. (c) When a resistor R is connected to a voltage generator v, the current i flowing in the circuit is computed from Ohm's Law.

resistor, namely voltage (v), current (i), and resistance (R). These quantities are not independent of one another, but their relationship is described by *Ohm's Law* which states that *the voltage across any resistor is equal to the current through the resistor times its resistance.* Mathematically, this is expressed as

Ohm's Law: *voltage = current × resistance*, i.e.,

$$v = i \times R .$$

After some algebraic manipulation, the following equations are also true:

$$i = \frac{v}{R} \quad \text{and} \quad R = \frac{v}{i} .$$

For example, with reference to the circuit in Figure 3.1(c), when 100 V are applied to a 50 Ω resistor, the value of the current is computed as $i = \frac{v}{R} = \frac{100\ V}{50\ \Omega} = 2\ A$.

3.2.6   Connecting Resistors in Series

When two or more resistors R_1, R_2, ... are connected end-to-end as in Figure 3.2(a), they are said to be connected *in series*. It can be shown that, in such an arrangement, the total resistance R_{tot} is given by the sum of the partial resistances, i.e.,

$$R_{tot} = R_1 + R_2 + \cdots .$$

For instance, in a circuit of four resistors $R_1 = 1\ \Omega$, $R_2 = 2\ \Omega$, $R_3 = 3\ \Omega$, and $R_4 = 4\ \Omega$ connected in series the total resistance is $R_{tot} = 1\ \Omega + 2\ \Omega + 3\ \Omega + 4\ \Omega = 10\ \Omega$.

In the particular case that there are N identical resistors R connected in series, the total resistance R_{tot} is given by

$$R_{tot} = N \times R .$$

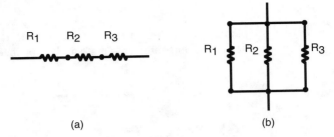

Figure 3.2   Example of resistors connected (a) in series and (b) in parallel.

As a second example, let us connect the same four resistors just considered to a voltage generator, as shown in Figure 3.3. This circuit, known as *voltage divider,*

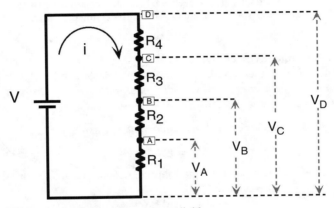

Figure 3.3   A simple circuit known as voltage divider.

can be used to control, for example, the *sensitivity* of a recording system (see Section 3.8.3). Considering that the current i flowing in the circuit is the same in all components, its value is computed by dividing the voltage by the total resistance, i.e.,

$$i = \frac{v}{R_{\text{tot}}} = \frac{40\ V}{10\ \Omega} = 4\ A\ .$$

The voltage at different points in the circuit can be computed from Ohm's Law, as follows:

Point A: $v_A = i \times R_1 = 4\ A \times 1\ \Omega = 4\ V$

Point B: $v_B = i \times (R_1 + R_2) = 4\ A \times 3\ \Omega = 12\ V$

Point C: $v_C = i \times (R_1 + R_2 + R_3) = 4\ A \times 6\ \Omega = 24\ V$

Point D: $v_D = i \times (R_1 + R_2 + R_3 + R_4) = 4\ A \times 10\ \Omega = 40\ V\ .$

Thus, in the case of neurophysiological recordings, if the generator v represents EEG activity, the user may select (by setting the appropriate sensitivity value) to amplify the full strength of the signal or part of it, depending on the signal's characteristics. In any case, it is important to note that the voltage at all points is proportional to v.

3.2.7   *Connecting Resistors in Parallel*

When the two ends of two or more resistors $R_1, R_2, \ldots$ are connected together as in Figure 3.2(b), the resistors are said to be connected *in parallel.* It can be shown that, in that case, the total resistance R_{tot} is given by

$$\frac{1}{R_{\text{tot}}} = \frac{1}{R_1} + \frac{1}{R_2} + \cdots .$$

In particular, when there are N identical resistors R connected in parallel, the total resistance R_{tot} is given by:

$$\frac{1}{R_{\text{tot}}} = \underbrace{\frac{1}{R} + \frac{1}{R} + \cdots}_{N \text{ times}} = N \times \frac{1}{R} = \frac{N}{R} \Rightarrow R_{\text{tot}} = \frac{R}{N} .$$

Notice that in this case, the total value is less than the value of each resistor. In fact, if the four resistors $R_1 = 1\,\Omega$, $R_2 = 2\,\Omega$, $R_3 = 3\,\Omega$, and $R_4 = 4\,\Omega$ considered in the previous section are connected in parallel, the total resistance becomes

$$\frac{1}{R_{\text{tot}}} = \frac{1}{1\,\Omega} + \frac{1}{2\,\Omega} + \frac{1}{3\,\Omega} + \frac{1}{4\,\Omega} = \frac{1}{2.08\,\Omega} \Rightarrow R_{\text{tot}} = 0.48\,\Omega .$$

3.2.8   *Capacitors and Inductors*

A *capacitor* consists of two conducting surfaces (plates) separated by an insulating material. When connected to a battery, this device can store energy in the form of electrical charge. That is, even when disconnected from the battery, a capacitor presents a potential difference between its plates, until it is discharged. In electronic circuits, capacitors are used to block the flow of direct current while allowing alternating current to pass.

An *inductor* can be obtained by inserting a permanent magnet into a coil. Movement of the magnet with respect to the coil induces an electromotive force in the coil that results in electrical current.

Several electrical components of specific value can be arranged in certain sequences to manipulate voltage or current in an electrical circuit, and they play a significant role in the design of EEG instrumentation. In particular, capacitors and resistors are especially important in the design of amplifiers and filters, which are discussed in Sections 3.6 and 4.4.1, respectively.

3.2.9   *Impedance*

In general, when resistors, capacitors, and inductors are connected to a voltage source, there is some opposition to the flow of current: resistors have *resistance,* while capacitors and inductors have *reactance.* The former is due to the molecular structure of the conductor itself, while the latter results from the time required to charge and discharge a capacitor, and from the field generated inside an inductor. *Impedance* denotes the combined effect of all three elements, and it is used only in connection with alternating currents. However, the term is often used in a general sense, even for circuits that may have only resistance.

It should be noted that in EEG instrumentation theory, there are at least three different measures of impedance: (1) the impedance of the electrodes, discussed in Section 3.3.1; (2) the input impedance of an amplifier, discussed in Section 3.7.3; and (3) the impedance of a filter, discussed in Section 4.4.5.

3.3   Electrodes

Electrical stimulation is delivered through stimulation of electrodes, which come in different types, sizes, and forms. Selection of the appropriate electrode type and its correct placement will determine the efficiency of stimulus delivery and affect the characteristics of the activity elicited.

On the other hand, the link between the generators of bioelectrical activity and the recording equipment is made by the recording electrodes, through which the ion flow within the biological sources becomes electron flow in the recording apparatus. The characteristics of the electrode/tissue interface determine the quality of the recorded signals.

3.3.1   Electrode Characteristics

Surface electrodes are placed on the skin using an *electrolyte,* a conductive jelly which, along with the body fluids, forms a layer of free chloride ions (Cl^-). When an electrode (which is practically a piece of metal) is placed in an electrolyte, two layers of electrical charges are formed: one on the surface of the electrode, and one of opposite charges on the electrolyte. A similar situation is generated at the skin-electrolyte junction. These double-layer formations are equivalent to a charged capacitor. Thus, at the electrode-electrolyte-skin interface a bias voltage develops (as if there was a battery).

Different metals develop different voltages when immersed in the same electrolyte. Therefore, when recording electrophysiological activity, it is imperative that the two electrodes of each recording channel be identical, so that the voltages developed at the skin-electrolyte interface are identical at the two electrodes. In that case, when these electrodes are connected to the inputs of a differential amplifier (see Section 3.7) the overall effect on the output signal will be zero. Otherwise, two dissimilar electrodes will form a constant voltage difference at the amplifier input, which will cause a baseline drift in the output and distort the recorded signals. In practice, however, there is always some variability, which causes real electrodes to present a certain amount of noise.

From the above, it is obvious that the overall impedance of an electrode, in addition to a purely resistive element, has also a capacitive component. The presence of the capacitive component will result in impedance changes which are a function of the frequency content of the recorded signal. Figure 3.4 depicts a simplified equivalent circuit of an electrode placed in electrolyte. The resistor R_s represents the overall

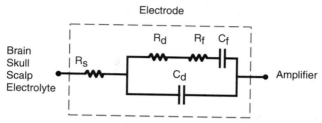

Figure 3.4   Equivalent circuit of a recording electrode placed in electrolyte.

resistance of the body fluid, skin, and electrolyte jelly; C_d and R_d are the resistive and capacitive components of the double layers; and finally C_f and R_f are frequency-dependents components. In general, an electrode presents higher impedance to low frequency signals, and vice versa.

The values of the various elements in the equivalent circuit of Figure 3.4 will depend on the material of the electrode. Typical EEG recordings are made with silver-silver chloride (AgAgCl) or gold-plated electrodes which minimize unwanted effects.

3.4   Types of Stimulation Electrodes

Several types of stimulation electrodes are depicted in Figure 3.5, including (a) metal bars, self-adhesive disposable, (b) disks, (c) tabs, (d) needles, and metal probes, which can be (e) monopolar or bipolar, with (f) straight or (g) hooked tips.

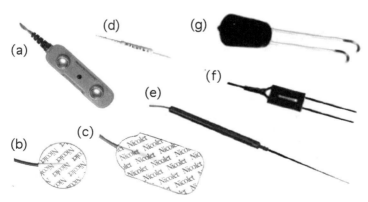

Figure 3.5   Different types of electrodes used for electrical stimulation.

To record somatosensory EPs, electrical stimuli can be delivered to a peripheral nerve from the skin surface using metal bars, self-adhesive disks, or sterile subdermal needles. The latter may have an advantage because they are easy to use and, since they get closer to the nerve than surface electrodes, the current necessary to elicit a response is much less. However, there is always the risk of an infection at the needle site, or of causing local skin damage if a stimulus of very high intensity is used.

Electrical stimulation of an exposed nerve or nerve root typically requires a sterilized bipolar or monopolar electrode consisting of an insulated metal probe with its distal tip exposed. Occasionally, specially designed "hook" electrodes that can wrap around a nerve are used.

3.5   Types of Recording Electrodes

Various types of recording electrodes are depicted in Figure 3.6. With reference to Figure 3.6, brain activity can be obtained using metal cup (a) or hypodermal needle (g) and corkscrew (b) electrodes. In general, needles are preferred in the operating room because they are easier to place (no collodion needed) and they maintain stable impedances over the course of several hours (no electrolyte to dry out). Again, however, there is the risk of an infection at the needle site.

Recordings from face and body muscles and from peripheral nerves outside the surgical field are obtained using needle electrodes, Figure 3.6(f)–(h), the size of which will depend on the depth of the structure to be monitored from the surface. In certain cases, hook electrodes are used to record the activity of an exposed nerve in the surgical field.

Stick-on electrodes are disposable disks or tabs shown in Figure 3.6(c) and (d), respectively, are very common also for recording, typically from hairless body areas, such as the popliteal fossa behind the leg (see Section 7.3.6), and Erb's point in the shoulder (see Section 7.3.5). A larger self-adhesive plate, Figure 3.6(e), is used for patient ground (see Section 3.5.1), since its large area guarantees a low impedance.

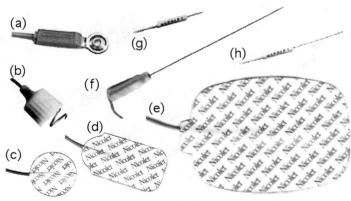

Figure 3.6   Different types of electrodes used for recording neurophysiological activity.

3.5.1   Patient Setup

Recording neurophysiological signals requires two electrodes connected to the input of an amplifier, one *active* and one for *reference*. Together, the amplifier and the two electrodes form a *recording channel*. Active electrodes are placed close to the structures at risk, whereas the reference electrode is placed at an indifferent location.

The common electrical connection for the electrical circuitry of the recording equipment is called the *ground*, and all voltages and impedances are measured with reference to it. A patient is also connected to this point through a large self-adhesive plate electrode, which is usually placed between the stimulation site and the first recording electrode. A typical location for the ground is the patient's shoulder.

All recording electrodes are attached to the amplifiers through a *head box*, the main function of which is to protect the recording system against interference during the use of the *electrocautery*[2] by limiting the amount of current flowing from the patient to the amplifiers. It can also serve as a selector for switching among different electrode groups, depending on the needs of the different phases of an operation.

An additional *isolation device*, typically internal to the amplifier box, is used for patient protection against electrical shock in case of equipment malfunction.

3.5.2   Placement of Stimulation Electrodes

Electrode location should be optimized so that electrical stimuli are delivered at a maximum efficiency, that is, all of the neuronal axons are forced to fire, while using the minimum current intensity. Electrodes should be placed over a nerve, approximately 2.5 cm apart, as shown in Figure 3.7. To obtain optimal stimulation, it is very important that the negative electrode, where the pulses of current are generated, be placed *proximally* or closer to the recording site.

At resting conditions, before the application of a stimulus, the inside of the nerve cell is negative with respect to the outside. During the application of a stimulus, negative charges accumulate under the negative electrode and depolarize the axonal membrane, resulting in an *action potential* traveling in both directions along the nerve fibers. Similarly, under the positive electrode accumulate large numbers of positive charges which simply hyperpolarize the membrane. The pulse moving toward the recoding site is strong enough to depolarize adjacent membrane patches which, typically, are at resting potential. However, the pulse moving in the opposite direction, or away from the recoding site, will have to overcome the large hyperpolarization potential established under the positive electrode in order to depolarize the membrane. Thus, when the positive electrode is placed in the pathway of the pulse, the effective amplitude of the stimulus is drastically decreased and, therefore, the efficiency of stimulation reduced.

---

[2]The *electrocautery* or *bovie* is a surgical device that employs high-voltage radiofrequency signals for cutting and coagulation.

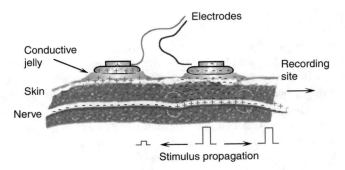

Figure 3.7 The negative electrode is placed proximally (closer to the recording site) for optimal stimulus delivery.

3.5.3   Placement of Recording Electrodes

Most laboratories use the internationally recognized 10–20 system for electrode placement, which uses 21 electrodes [26], but it can be extended to include additional ones, as needed. The location of the electrodes is shown in Figure 3.8. The system is based

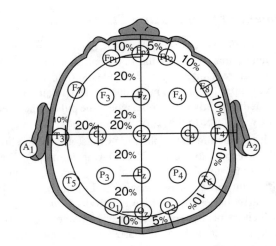

Figure 3.8 Location of the electrodes used in the internationally recognized 10-20 electrode placement system.

on measurements from four standard bony landmarks on the head, namely the nasion, the inion, and the left and right pre-auricular points. The location of the various electrodes is either 10 or 20% of the distance between two landmarks. Also, all odd-numbered electrodes are on the left, while the even-numbered ones are on the right.

For proper placement of conventional cup EEG electrodes, the skin is first cleaned and prepared with an abrasive paste which reduces scalp resistance by removing oils and dead cells. Then, the electrode is secured on the skin with collodion (a kind of glue). Finally, the electrode is filled with a conductive jelly, which facilitates ion movement from the skin to the electrode and lowers the skin impedance. Alternatively, a water-soluble conductive paste can be used for electrode attachment to the scalp. Correct skin preparation before electrode placement allows for a small impedance and low signal distortion over the entire range of clinically useful frequencies.

For self-adhesive disposable electrodes, the skin is first cleaned with alcohol and then the tabs, which are already pre-treated with conductive jelly, are applied and secured in place with surgical tape.

Sterile needle electrodes are placed under the surface of the scalp, in areas that have been disinfected with alcohol, and they are held in place with surgical tape. In cases where excessive maneuvering of the patient's head is expected, needles can be secured in place with sterile surgical staples.

3.5.4 *Montages*

The term *montage* refers to the particular combination of electrodes examined at a given time. In general, there are two kinds of montages, bipolar, and referential.

In a *bipolar* montage each channel involves the recording between two active scalp electrodes. These montages typically include chains running anteroposteriorly or transversely, using the same linkage over both hemispheres [12].

In a *referential* montage, on the other hand, each channel involves the recording between an active electrode and an "inactive" one, known as the *reference*. Theoretically, the reference is completely silent and has a zero potential. In practice, however, all locations on the head are active to some degree, so electrodes are referred to less active locations, such as the ears. Figure 3.9 shows two very common montages, a bipolar one, known also as "double banana," and another one which is referential.

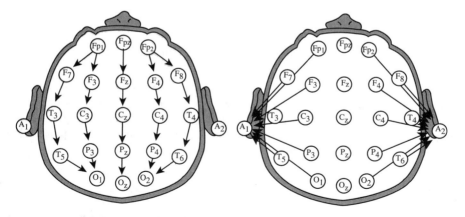

Figure 3.9 Two very common montages used for recording EEG. The montage on the left is bipolar, while the one on the right is referential.

3.6   Amplifiers

The heart of every recording system consists of a set of amplifiers. Figure 3.10(a) shows a schematic diagram of a *single-ended amplifier,* which has three terminals: an *input,* an *output,* and a *ground.*[3] Figure 3.10(b) depicts another common representation equivalent to the first one. The input and output voltages are measured with respect to the ground.

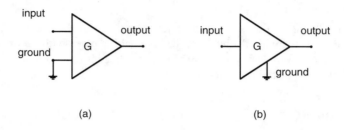

(a)   (b)

Figure 3.10   Schematic diagram of single-ended amplifiers: (a) and (b) two equivalent representations.

The *gain G* of an amplifier refers to the amount of amplification provided, and it is defined as the ratio of the output voltage v_{out} to the input voltage v_{in}, i.e.,

$$G = \frac{v_{\text{out}}}{v_{\text{in}}} .$$

Thus, if the output voltage of an amplifier is 20 mV when the input voltage is 0.2 mV, then the amplifier's gain is

$$G = \frac{20\ mV}{0.2\ mV} = 100 .$$

Notice that gain has no units: since it is defined as a ratio of voltages, the units cancel out.

Certain amplifiers, in addition to amplifying the input signal, they also invert its polarity, and for this reason they are called *inverting* amplifiers. Therefore, the overall effect is a negative gain. The two types of amplifiers are schematically shown in Figure 3.11. For example, a signal of 1 mV at the input of an inverting amplifier with gain 100 would result in an output signal of -100 mV.

---

[3]More properly, the ground terminal should be referred to as *neutral,* since practically it is never connected directly to the earth ground.

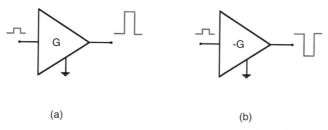

(a)   (b)

Figure 3.11   Schematic diagram of (a) a noninverting and (b) an inverting amplifier.

3.7 *Differential Amplifiers*

3.7.1 **Basic Operation**

Two single-ended amplifiers of the same gain, one of which is noninverting and the other inverting, can be connected together to form a *differential* amplifier. Figure 3.12(a) shows a conceptual procedure for constructing such a device, while Figure 3.12(b) shows a more common equivalent representation. A differential am-

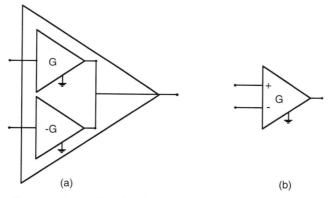

(a)   (b)

Figure 3.12   Conceptual procedure for obtaining a differential amplifier.

plifier has two inputs, called *input 1* and *input 2,* one output, and a ground. Again, the voltages at input 1, input 2, and output, are measured with reference to the ground.

The output of a differential amplifier is proportional only to the voltage *difference* present at the two inputs. To see this, let us consider the case where a signal of 2 mV is applied to input 1 (noninverting input) and a signal of 5 mV is applied to input 2 (inverting input). If the gain of the amplifier is, say, 100, then the output signal will be equal to

$$\underbrace{2\,mV \times 100}_{\text{input 1}} + \underbrace{5\,mV \times (-100)}_{\text{input 2}} = \underbrace{200\,mV - 500\,mV}_{\text{output}} = -300\,mV \ .$$

On the other hand, if we take the difference between the signals at input 1 and input

2 and then we amplify it 100 times, we obtain the same result, i.e.,

$$(2\,mV - 5\,mV) \times 100 = -3\,mV \times 100 = -300\,mV \ .$$

Thus, the basic operation of a differential amplifier is to subtract the voltage at input 2 from that at input 1 and to amplify only the voltage difference.

3.7.2   *Need for Differential Amplifiers*

From the above example, it would seem that the differential amplifier could be replaced by a simple single-ended amplifier. However, there are at least two reasons why single-ended amplifiers cannot be used in EEG recordings.

The first reason can be explained with reference to Figure 3.13. Let us say we want to record EEG from multiple areas of the scalp simultaneously, using a bipolar parasagittal montage (such as the "double banana" depicted in Figure 3.9) and single-ended amplifiers as shown in Figure 3.13(a). Then, we will have to connect the F_{p1}

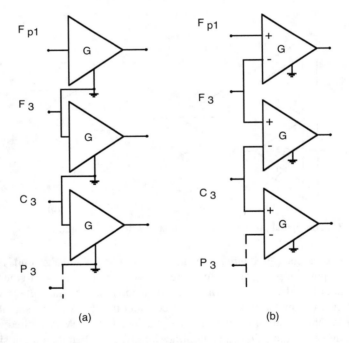

(a)   (b)

Figure 3.13   Use of (a) single-ended and (b) differential amplifiers for bipolar recording of neurophysiological signals.

and F_3 leads to the input and ground, respectively, of the first amplifier; F_3 and C_3 to input and ground of the second amplifier; C_3 and P_3 to input and ground of the third amplifier, and so on. Under this arrangement though, the input of each amplifier is effectively connected to the ground of the previous one (except for the first amplifier) and, therefore, the inputs of *all* amplifiers (except for the first one) are connected to ground. As a result, all output signals will be zero. On the contrary, if we use differential amplifiers for the same bipolar montage, as in Figure 3.13(b), the inputs will not be grounded and we will be able to get the desired recordings.

The second reason for using differential amplifiers to record neurophysiological activity, such as the EEG, stems from the observation that when the same voltage is applied to both inputs, the amplifier's output is zero. This is known as *common mode rejection*. Interference signals, such as the omnipresent 60 Hz noise from the power lines, most likely will affect equally both inputs of a differential amplifier and, therefore, they will have a zero total effect on the output. Thus, the output of a differential amplifier theoretically is noise-free and represents only neurophysiological activity. This last statement is true only when certain conditions that are described in Section 3.7.5 are met.

3.7.3   Amplifier Input Impedance

Every amplifier is characterized by its *internal input impedance R*. Although the actual electronic circuit is very complicated, the input impedance of an amplifier can be conceptualized as a resistor R connected between the input and the ground.

Figure 3.14 shows a schematic diagram of a differential amplifier where the internal impedance of each input is shown explicitly. When an external generator is connected

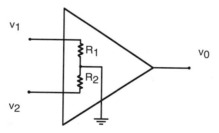

Figure 3.14   Internal input impedance R_1 and R_2 of a differential amplifier.

to an amplifier input, current i flows to the ground through the electrode and the internal resistor, and the voltage v developed at that input is equal to the voltage drop across the internal resistor R. This voltage can be computed from *Ohm's Law* as $v = i \times R$ (see Section 3.2.5).

3.7.4   Amplifier Performance

Ideally, a differential amplifier should amplify only the difference between the signals present at the two inputs, and reject all signals common to both inputs. For example, when recording EEG, it should amplify the difference between, say, a frontal and a central channel and, at the same time, reject the large ECG signal common to both channels. Since the desired signal is the differential voltage, amplification of the common-mode signal produces an error at the output that is indistinguishable from the signal.

To understand the behavior of a differential amplifier, its overall gain is typically computed under two distinct conditions: (1) with a small differential signal, like the EEG, applied to the inputs; this is called the *differential gain*; and (2) with a relatively large signal, like a power line interference, applied equally to both inputs; this is called the *common mode gain*.

The performance of the amplifier is then measured by the so-called *common mode rejection ratio* (CMRR) defined as the ratio of the differential gain over the common mode gain, i.e.,

$$\text{CMRR} = \frac{\text{differential gain}}{\text{common mode gain}} .$$

Typical CMRR values for a good EEG amplifier are 10,000:1 or even 20,000:1. A loose interpretation of a CMRR of 10,000:1 is the following: *for every 10,000 "units" of common signals that affect input 1 and input 2 equally, only 1 "unit" will be amplified, while the rest will be rejected.*

Often the CMRR is given in *decibels* (dB). A number can be converted to decibels by first taking the logarithm in base 10 of the number and then multiplying by 20, i.e.,

$$\text{CMRR}_{\text{dB}} = 20 \times \log_{10}(\text{CMRR}) .$$

Thus, a CMRR of 1000:1 is 60 dB, since $\log_{10}(1000) = 3$ and $20 \times 3 = 60$. Similarly, a CMRR of 10,000:1 is 80 dB, while 100,000:1 is 100 dB.

3.7.5 *Optimal Recordings*

The following two requirements are necessary for obtaining high quality recordings:

1. All electrode impedances must be low. An intuitive explanation for this requirement can be obtained using the diagram in Figure 3.15 which shows an over-simplified electrical equivalent circuit of a single-channel recording system.

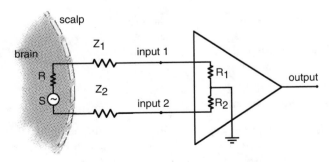

Figure 3.15   Simplified equivalent circuit of a single-channel recording system.

The amplifier inputs are connected to a subject's head through two electrodes of impedance Z_1 and Z_2, respectively. In this diagram, S indicates a hypothetical generator of brain activity, whereas R accounts for the resistance of all tissues underlying the electrodes, namely the brain, skull, and scalp. Ideally, there should be no resistance in the circuit outside the amplifier, so that the voltage at the amplifier input equals that of the generator inside the brain. In reality, though, part of the signal will be lost in the impedances of the tissues (R) and electrodes (Z_1 and Z_2), and this loss must be kept to a minimum.

Ohm's Law states that the voltage drop across a resistor is proportional to (1) the current i through it and (2) the impedance R (voltage = current × impedance). Thus, to minimize signal loss we must (1) minimize the current flowing in the circuit, and (2) minimize the value of all external impedances. For the first requirement, we know that by design the amplifier's input impedances R_1 and R_2 are very large (typically around 10 MΩ or more). Thus, the current flowing in the external circuit is indeed kept very low. For the second requirement, there is nothing we can do to minimize the impedance R inside the head. Therefore, only the electrode impedances Z_1 and Z_2 can be controlled and this is why they should be kept very small (usually less than 2 kΩ).

Another reason for maintaining small impedances is that electrodes act like antennas: the higher their impedance, the higher the noise they pick up from radiating fields, such as those generated by power lines.

2. All electrode impedances must be identical. This can be illustrated using the arrangement in Figure 3.16, which represents a hypothetical interference signal S applied to both inputs of a differential amplifier through two electrodes of impedance Z_1 and Z_2, respectively.

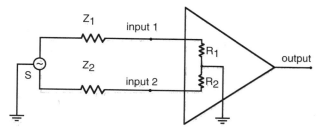

Figure 3.16   Common mode signal rejection of a differential amplifier.

The impedance seen now at each input is the sum $Z_1 + R_1$ in the upper branch, and the sum $Z_2 + R_2$ in the lower branch. By design, R_1 and R_2 are identical. Thus, if the electrode impedances Z_1 and Z_2 are also equal, the total impedance in the two input circuits are equal. In that case, from Ohm's Law, the currents flowing in the two branches are the same, and the voltages v_1 and v_2 at input 1 and input 2 are equal. And, since the two input voltages are equal, the output of the differential amplifier will be zero.

When the electrode impedances are identical, the amplifier is said to be *balanced.* In that case, the amplifier functions properly and rejects interference signals (noise) that are common to both inputs. Otherwise, an impedance difference will allow part of the noise to be amplified, and the resulting erroneous output signal will be proportional to the amplifier's gain, which can be in the order of tens of thousands.

3.7.6   Effects of Imbalances

As mentioned earlier, a differential amplifier is nothing more than two single-ended amplifiers having the same gain, one of which is also inverting. The performance of a differential amplifier depends *critically* on the assumption that the gains of the two amplifiers are exactly matched (except, of course, for the sign). In reality, slight variations exist mainly because of imbalances in the input impedances.

To understand the effects of a variation, let us consider an example in which the gain of one input is slightly off, say by only 1%, and let us compute first the differential gain and then the common mode gain. Also, let us assume that the noninverting input (input 1) has a gain of 100, whereas the inverting input (input 2) has a gain of −99. If we apply a small signal of −2 μV at input 1 and +8 μ V at input 2, as shown in Figure 3.17, the output signal will be equal to

$$\underbrace{-2\ \mu V \times 100}_{\text{input 1}} + \underbrace{8\ \mu V \times (-99)}_{\text{input 2}} = -200\ \mu V - 792\ \mu V = -992\ \mu V \ .$$

Thus, when a −10 μV differential signal is applied between the two inputs, it is

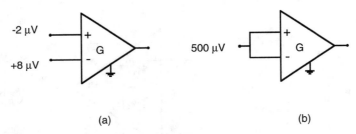

(a)   (b)

Figure 3.17   Example of computing the CMRR.

amplified to −992 μV, and the overall gain is 99.2 instead of 100. Thus, in this case the effect of the imbalance is practically negligible.

Let us now apply a larger signal of +500 μV, which would represent a typical interference signal in the operating room, equally to both inputs. In this case, the output will be

$$\underbrace{+500\ \mu V \times 100}_{\text{input 1}} + \underbrace{500\ \mu V \times (-99)}_{\text{input 2}} = 50{,}000\ \mu V - 49{,}500\ \mu V = 500\ \mu V \ .$$

Interestingly, the output is *not zero,* as it should be. The amplifier gain in this case is 1. Thus, the amplifier lost its ability to reject signals that are common to both inputs. Therefore, when this large interference signal of 500 μV hits the amplifier it will appear at the output, and it will obliterate the smaller EEG signal.

In our example, the CMRR of the amplifier is approximately 40 dB, which is far below the more typical value of 60 dB.

3.7.7 The Balanced Amplifier

From the above discussion we can conclude that the first requirement of low impedance is more important, since low impedances not only minimize signal loss, but they also keep the amplifier close to being balanced.

Indeed, by design, the input impedances R_1 and R_2 of an amplifier are identical and have a very large value. When an electrode of impedance Z_1 is connected to input 1, the total impedance $R_{1,\text{tot}}$ is given by the sum of the two impedances, i.e., $R_{1,\text{tot}} = Z_1 + R_1$. Similarly, $R_{2,\text{tot}} = Z_2 + R_2$. If Z_1 and Z_2 are small compared to R_1 and R_2, respectively, then $R_{1,\text{tot}}$ will be approximately equal to $R_{2,\text{tot}}$.

For example, say that $R_1 = R_2 = 20 \text{ M}\Omega = 20,000,000 \ \Omega$, while $Z_1 = 2,000 \ \Omega$ and $Z_2 = 1,500 \ \Omega$. Then, $R_{1,\text{tot}} = Z_1 + R_1 = 20,002,000 \ \Omega$, and $R_{2,\text{tot}} = Z_2 + R_2 = 20,001,500 \ \Omega$. We see that $R_{1,\text{tot}} \approx R_{2,\text{tot}}$. Thus, although Z_1 and Z_2 are not equal, the fact that they have low values allows the amplifier to remain balanced and reject unwanted signals common to both inputs.

3.7.8 *Multi-channel Referential Recordings*

In multi-channel referential recordings, where the same electrode is shared by several amplifiers, some imbalance can result even when individual electrodes have equal impedances. An example of such a situation is depicted in Figure 3.18, where the same electrode Fz is shared by two amplifiers, A and B.

In this case, the R_2 impedances of the common input (input 2) are effectively connected in parallel, at one end through the common electrode and at the other end through the ground. The equivalent total impedance at the common input is smaller than the individual impedances (see Section 3.2.7). Therefore, the two inputs of all amplifiers will be imbalanced, even though individual electrodes have the same impedance.

To avoid this effect, typical recording systems use specialized *preamplifiers* between the electrodes and the actual differential amplifiers. These devices present very high input impedance and very low output impedance. As a result, at the actual differential amplification stage the input impedances are balanced.

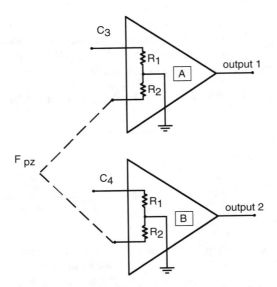

Figure 3.18 Input impedance imbalance in multi-channel referential recordings.

3.8 *Amplifier Characteristics*

3.8.1 *Polarity Convention*

As mentioned earlier, neurophysiological activity is recorded using differential amplifiers. In each channel the amplitude of the output signal is proportional to the voltage
difference between the electrode connected to input 1 and the electrode connected to
input 2. If there is no difference in the input voltages the amplifier's output is zero,
and this corresponds to the *baseline*. In effect, the amplifier measures the activity
of one electrode with respect to the activity of another electrode. Both electrodes
may detect activity of the same polarity (positive or negative) but one of the two
may be less positive or less negative than the other one. Hence, the polarity of the
measurement depends on the choice of reference, that is, whether input 1 or input 2
is considered to be the reference. Typically, polarity is determined by following the
"negative up" convention: if the value voltage at input 1 minus voltage at input 2 is
negative the displayed output activity is above the baseline, and vice versa, as depicted in Figure 3.19. For example, according to this convention, if a constant signal
of -50 μV is applied to input 1 and a constant signal of -20 μV is applied to input 2
(both measured with respect to ground) then the displayed activity will be a flat line
30 μV above the baseline, measuring a voltage difference of -30 μV.

3.8.2 *Dynamic Range*

The range of input voltages over which an amplifier is linear, that is, the output
voltage is proportional to the input, is called the amplifier's *dynamic range*. If the
input voltage is less than the minimum value in the range, the output voltage will be

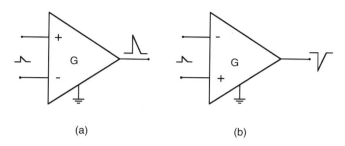

Figure 3.19   Polarity convention for (a) noninverting and (b) inverting differential amplifiers.

zero, whereas if the input voltage is larger than the maximum value in the range, the amplifier's output will *saturate,* reaching its maximum value. Any further increase in the input will result in the same output voltage. Thus, outside the dynamic range of the amplifier, the output cannot follow the input.

3.8.3   *Sensitivity*

The *sensitivity* of an amplifier is the minimum input voltage difference necessary to produce a nonzero output signal. Values below that minimum level are considered "noise" and they have no effect on the output signal. The sensitivity of an amplifier will also determine what input values cover its entire dynamic range. If the sensitivity is very high, a small input value will result in a large output signal, and a slight further increase will force the amplifier to reach the maximum of its dynamic range.

In EEG applications however, amplifier sensitivity refers to the *displayed signal sensitivity,* which simply controls the scale of a trace on paper or on the computer screen. That is, it dictates how many millimeters on the display correspond to one microvolt in the output, and makes plots look bigger or smaller.

Thus, the *sensitivity* can be defined as *the amplitude of the input voltage required to produce a 1 mm deflection in the recorded trace.* Sensitivity is usually measured in μV/mm. The input voltage V, the output trace A, and the sensitivity S are related through the following formula:

$$S = \frac{V}{A} .$$

After some algebraic manipulation, the following equations are also true:

$$A = \frac{V}{S} \quad \text{and} \quad V = S \times A .$$

As an example, let us consider a conventional EEG machine where the pens have a total range of motion of approximately 35 mm. Thus, a sensitivity of 7 μV/mm will give a total output range of 245 μV, whereas a sensitivity of 2 μV/mm will give an range of only 70 μV. So, if one is interested in detecting small input variations (such as, for example, activity on a facial muscle) a high sensitivity must be used (e.g., 1 μV/mm). Conversely, if one is interested in detecting big events only (such as, for example, epileptogenic spikes), a lower sensitivity is much more adequate, otherwise there is the risk that signals will be clipped, and thus, data will be lost.

3.8.4   *Signal-to-Noise Ratio*

The *signal-to-noise ratio* in a recording refers to the ratio of the amplitude of neurophysiological activity (the signal) to the amplitude of the interference (the noise). One way to improve it is by appropriate adjustment of the amplifier's sensitivity. For instance, when recording evoked potentials, activity that exceeds 100 μV can be safely considered of noncerebral origin—it could be muscle activity, or electrical interference—and thus should be rejected. However, if the sensitivity is too high a large number of single trials are rejected; if it is too low, the recordings are contaminated by large amounts of noise. As a rule of thumb, in the case of evoked potentials the sensitivity should be such that approximately 10% of the single trials are rejected.

3.9   *Review Questions*

1. What are the various components of a recording system adequate for intraoperative monitoring (IOM).

2. What kind of stimuli are used to elicit evoked responses?

3. Give examples of different kinds of stimulation electrodes and explain their specific use.

4. When recording SEPs, stimulating electrodes are placed so that the negative electrode is closer to the recording site. Explain why.

5. Draw the equivalent circuit of an electrode placed in electrolyte, and explain the meaning of the various components.

6. What is the relationship between the impedance of the recording electrode and the frequency of the recorded signals.

7. Does the use of needle electrodes in the OR have an advantage over, say, bar electrodes? Explain.

8. What is the main function of an amplifier?

9. Draw a diagram of a single-ended amplifier and identify its major parts.

10. How is the gain of an amplifier defined?

11. The voltage at the output of an amplifier with gain 80 is 160 μV. What is the value of the corresponding input voltage?

12. What would be the output of an inverting amplifier with gain 100 when the input is 2 mv?

13. Draw a diagram of a differential amplifier.

14. Describe in one sentence the function performed by a differential amplifier.

15. A differential amplifier has an overall gain of 1000. What is the value of the output voltage when a signed of 2 mV is applied to the noninverting input while at the inverting input is applied to a signal of 1 mV?

16. Is it possible to obtain bipolar EEG recordings using single-ended amplifiers? Justify your answer.

17. When you record EEG between, say, F8 and C4, using a differential amplifier, do you expect to see any ECG activity at the output? Explain why.

18. Give Ohm's Law.

19. What is the input impedance of amplifier?

20. What are the two tasks that a differential amplifier has to accomplish simultaneously?

21. What is the quantity that measures the performance of a differential amplifier, and how is it defined?

22. What are the two requirements for optimal recordings?

23. Explain why the impedance of the recording electrodes must be low.

24. What does it mean for an amplifier to be balanced?

25. Explain why all recording electrodes must have identical impedances?

26. What is the main effect of an imbalanced amplifier?

27. Two resistors, $R_1 = 1\ \Omega$ and $R_2 = 2\ k\Omega$, are connected first in series and then in parallel. What is the value of total resistance R_{tot} in each case?

28. What kind of effect do referential recordings have on an amplifier's input impedance?

29. What is the typical polarity convention used with evoked potential recordings?

30. What is the dynamic range of an amplifier?

31. What is the sensitivity of a differential amplifier?

32. Define displayed signal sensitivity in conventional EEG recordings.

33. In which case would you use higher sensitivity settings in your amplifier, when recording beta activity or when recording ECG?

34. How is the signal-to-noise ratio defined?

35. What is the rule of thumb for selecting the amplifier sensitivity when recording EPs?

chapter 4

Electrophysiological Recordings

4.1 Introduction

Neurophysiological recordings provide a reliable way to monitor the functional integrity of the nervous system during the course of surgery. Proper interpretation of the recorded signals, however, requires understanding of certain simple signal characteristics, such as amplitude and frequency content. Also essential is the familiarity with simple forms of processing, such as filtering and averaging, that these signals must undergo before their relevant features can be extracted. Only then continuous analysis of the various patterns of activity, and of their evolution over time, will allow the identification of clinically significant changes.

4.2 Signal Characteristics

4.2.1 Amplitude

The *amplitude* of a signal, such as the EEG, refers to the magnitude of the vertical extend describing the activity at a particular point in time, and it is measured in volts (V).[1]

Amplitude represents the voltage difference between a point in the signal and the *baseline,* which is a reference representing zero amplitude at the output of a differential amplifier. Recall that zero amplitude means that signals of the same amplitude are applied to both inputs. In the example of Figure 4.1, the arbitrary signal $x(t)$ at time 1 msec has an amplitude of 3.2 V, while at time 6 msec its amplitude drops to about 1.9 V.

4.2.2 Frequency

With reference to a pure sinusoidal signal, *frequency* is defined in hertz (Hz), and simply denotes the number of signal oscillations (or cycles) per second. For example, the signal $x(t)$ in Figure 4.2(a) exhibits two cycles in each one-second interval, so its

---

[1]Typically, the amplitude of EEG activity is below 200 mV, while the amplitude of most evoked potential components can only reach a few μV.

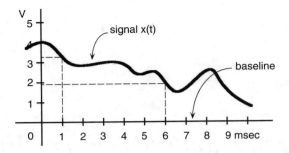

Figure 4.1 The amplitude of a signal $x(t)$ over time is measured with respect to the baseline.

frequency is 2 Hz. Similarly, the signal $y(t)$ in Figure 4.2(c) has a frequency of 3 Hz. However, its amplitude is half the amplitude of $x(t)$.

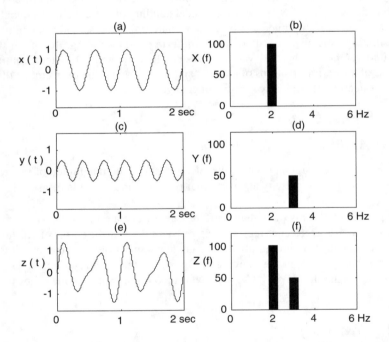

Figure 4.2 Sinusoidal signals in the time domain (left) and the corresponding spectra (right).

The above figures represent the signals $x(t)$ and $y(t)$ in the *time domain*, since they depict the signals' evolution over time. However, signals can also be represented in the *frequency domain*, where a special graph, called a *spectrogram*, shows the various frequency components (or spectrum) of a signal.

Figure 4.2(b) and Figure 4.2(d) show the spectra corresponding to the signals $x(t)$ and $y(t)$, respectively. Notice that both spectra are zero everywhere, except at the frequencies of 2 and 3 Hz, respectively. Additionally, since the amplitude of $x(t)$ is twice the amplitude of $y(t)$, this difference is also reflected on the height of the spectral bars.

The *duration* of a wave is the time it persists, and it is measured in seconds. The frequency of a specific wave can be determined by measuring its duration d in seconds, and then converting it into frequency by taking the inverse. In the example of Figure 4.2(a), each wave (a complete cycle) in the signal $x(t)$ has a duration $d = \frac{1}{2}$ sec. Thus its frequency is $f = \frac{1}{d} = \frac{1}{\frac{1}{2}} = 2$ Hz. Similarly, each wave in the signal $y(t)$ in Figure 4.2(c) has a duration $d = \frac{1}{3}$ sec and frequency $f = \frac{1}{d} = \frac{1}{\frac{1}{3}} = 3$ Hz.

The summation of two oscillatory signals is still oscillatory. Thus, the signal $z(t) = x(t) + y(t)$, obtained by summing $x(t)$ and $y(t)$, oscillates (Figure 4.2(e)), and its spectrum has two components at 2 and 3 Hz (Figure 4.2(f)).

A segment of neurophysiological activity is composed of many waves and several frequencies. In the case of EEG, and especially for rhythmic activity such as alpha, each wave corresponds to a complete cycle. Therefore, to compute the frequency content of a waveform, it is enough to count the number of waves contained in a 1 sec interval. Figure 4.3 depicts a sample of EEG which is about 2.3 sec long. The horizontal calibration bar indicates a 1 sec interval. In this example, the frequency of the various waves enclosed in the box is computed considering that waves 1, 2, and 3 have a duration of 0.075, 0.175, and 0.275 sec, respectively; thus, the corresponding frequencies are 13.3, 5.7, and 3.6 Hz, respectively.

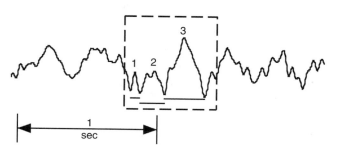

Figure 4.3 Example of computing the frequency of a specific component in a waveform.

4.3 Frequency Analysis

4.3.1 The Fourier Transform

In several cases, it is of interest to know the frequency content of a generic unknown signal. A more formal way to accomplish this is through *Fourier analysis,* typically using a Fast Fourier Transform (FFT) computer algorithm. In this technique, a signal is decomposed into a finite number of sinusoidal waves, each having different frequency and amplitude. The squared amplitude of each sinusoidal is proportional to the power of the signal at that frequency. Plotting these values against frequency produces an estimate of the *power spectrum* of the original signal.

Figure 4.4 shows a waveform which is 1 sec long, having maximum peak-to-peak amplitude of 9 μV. FFT analysis decomposes this signal into three sine waves having frequencies of 4, 7, and 11 Hz, and amplitude 12, 6, and 3 μV, respectively. Plotting the squared values of the magnitudes against frequency yields an estimate of the signal's power spectrum.

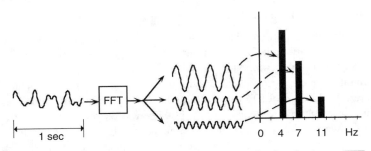

Figure 4.4   Procedure for estimating the power spectrum of a signal using an FFT.

4.3.2   *Time and Frequency Representation*

The original time series and its representation in the frequency domain are completely equivalent, in the sense that one can be obtained from the other through a mathematical transformation. That is, the original signal in the time domain can be reconstructed from its frequency domain representation by combining all of its frequency components using a mathematical operation called *inverse Fourier transform*. Thus, interpretation of an EEG recording in the frequency domain, which often is much easier than interpretation in the time domain, is equally valid.

4.3.3   *Computerized EEG Analysis*

Interpretation of a clinical EEG requires visual analysis from an expert (typically a neurologist) in order to extract the relevant features of the activity. The expert typically goes back and forth in the record in order to reliably identify clinically relevant patterns of activity. In the operating room, however, where interpretation must be performed in real time, reliable detection of any significant changes in amplitude or frequency content requires visual analysis of the current EEG trace and mental comparison of it with all the traces obtained previously. This challenging task can be alleviated through computerized EEG analysis, which offers several ways to process, compress, and display the EEG data more efficiently. The technique most commonly used during monitoring is frequency analysis.

As mentioned in Section 4.2.2, information regarding the amplitude and frequency content of a signal can be obtained from its power spectrum, which represents the distribution of signal power at each frequency. Long EEG recordings can be represented compactly in a *Compressed Spectral Array* (CSA) format.

The procedure for obtaining such a graph is schematically shown in Figures 4.5 and 4.6. First, the EEG is divided in several nonoverlapping segments, called *epochs.* Each epoch can represent, for example, 2 sec of EEG data. Then, the spectrum of each epoch is computed, using an FFT, and also *smoothed,* as shown in Figure 4.5. The smoothing operation removes the abrupt changes in the signal, so that the previously irregular jagged form of the signal now has a continuous appearance. Finally, the smoothed spectra of successive EEG epochs are plotted vertically, thus creating a pseudo-3-dimensional graph, as shown in Figure 4.6.

CSA graphs can clearly visualize the evolution in time of the dominant frequencies in the EEG data. For instance, in the example of Figure 4.6 one can clearly see a shift toward lower frequencies at time t_6 (arrow), since the highest peak around 10 Hz has decreased in amplitude, while the 5 Hz peak has increased.

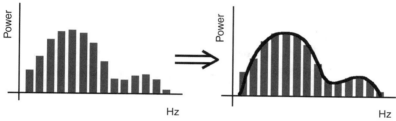

Figure 4.5   Procedure for constructing of smooth spectrum.

Different EEG monitoring systems use different representation techniques. For example, additional features, such as trend plots of peak power (i.e., plots of the frequency of the highest peak in the spectrum over time), spectral edge (i.e., plots of the value of the highest frequency in the spectrum over time), etc., may also be available.

4.4   Data Processing

All neurophysiological recordings contain noise which is due to extraneous biological activity, electrical interference, or it is inherent to instrumentation. In general, electrical noise and other interference signals generated in the operating room contain a random mixture of *all* frequencies, whereas neurophysiological activity contains only *specific* frequencies. Unfortunately, the frequency content of the "signal" and "noise" overlap. The use of some signal enhancement or noise reduction technique increases the *signal-to-noise ratio,* i.e., the amplitude of the signal compared to the amplitude of the noise. Two very common techniques for that purpose are filtering

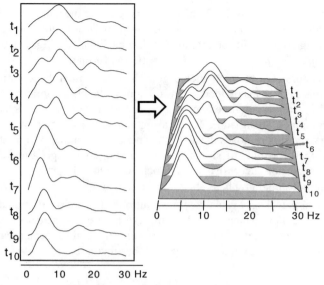

Figure 4.6   Procedure for constructing a CSA representation.

and averaging. The former is used for all kinds of activity, whether spontaneous or averaged, whereas the latter is obviously applied only to evoked responses.

4.4.1   Filtering

A *filter* is a device for attenuating certain frequency components in a recording, while leaving others unaffected. Neurophysiological recordings contain noise at low and high frequencies, and filters serve to remove *only* the part of noise that does not overlap with the signal by attenuating all signals outside the frequency range of interest.

Conventional recording systems employ three kinds of filters: low frequency, high frequency, and 60 Hz notch filters. *Low frequency filters* (LFF) reduce the amplitude of slow waves without attenuating faster waves. Similarly, *high frequency filters* (HFF) reduce the amplitude of fast waves while leaving slower waves intact.[2] A *notch* filter removes a narrow band of frequencies around 60 Hz, which is the main frequency of interference from power lines.

4.4.2   Frequency Response

The effects of a filter on a specific waveform may be inferred from the filter's *frequency response,* which is a graphical representation of the effects of the filter on the amplitude of individual frequencies. In such a graph, the horizontal axis represents frequency, while the vertical axis represents percentage of amplitude; alternatively, the vertical

---

[2]LFFs are also known as *highpass* filters, since high frequencies can pass through them unaffected. Similarly, HFFs are also known as *lowpass* filters.

axis may represent amplitude attenuation. Often, the frequency axis is not linear, but it is given in a logarithmic scale, in which case the distance between successive tick marks on the axis is not constant, but it follows a logarithmic progression. The overall effect of such a representation is a compression of the total length of the axis.

4.4.3 Low Frequency Filters (LFF)

Let us consider an example of LFF with cutoff frequency at 10 Hz. The dashed line in Figure 4.7 shows the frequency response of an *ideal* filter with a very sharp transition from full attenuation (0% amplitude) to no attenuation (100% amplitude): all frequencies below 10 Hz are attenuated to zero amplitude, while all frequencies above 10 Hz remain intact.

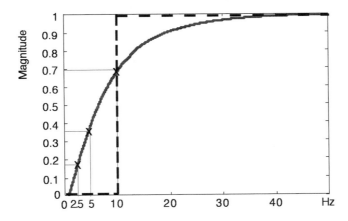

Figure 4.7 Frequency response of an ideal (dashed line) and real (solid line) LFF with cutoff frequency of 10 Hz.

In reality, though, filters are constructed using electronic components, mostly re-sistors and capacitors, which cannot be charged and discharged instantly, but they need a certain amount of time. Thus, real filters cannot follow such abrupt changes. As the solid line in Figure 4.7 shows, the frequency response of a real filter rises more smoothly. In that case, by definition the cutoff represents the frequency at which a 3 dB amplitude attenuation occurs, or the frequency at which the amplitude has been reduced to about 70% of the original value.[3] In our example, the amplitude of all frequency components of 10 Hz will be attenuated to about 70% of the original value.

To understand the rest of the frequency response curve, it can be shown that as the frequency is halved, the amplitude is reduced progressively by half. It is said that the curve has a slope of 6 dB/octave (-6 dB ≈ 0.5). Thus, in our example, at the

---

[3]Using the formula in Section 3.7.4, -3 dB $= 0.707 = 70.2\% \approx 70\%$.

frequency of 5 Hz the amplitude of all components will be attenuated to about 35% of the *original* value, at 2.5 Hz, it will be attenuated to only 1.75%, and so on. The final response of the filter can be approximated by plotting a smooth line connecting all these points and reaching the maximum amplitude.

4.4.4   High Frequency Filters (HFF)

Like the frequency response of a LFF, the frequency response of a HFF can help us understand what frequencies are attenuated by the filter and by how much.

As an example, Figure 4.8 shows the frequency response of a HFF filter with a cutoff frequency at 35 Hz. The *ideal* case is again shown with a dashed line, while the solid line with the smoother roll-off represents the response of a real filter. Again, the cutoff frequency of 35 Hz indicates that the amplitude of all components at that frequency will be attenuated to about 70% of the original value.

For the rest of the frequency response curve, it can be shown that as the frequency doubles, the amplitude of frequency components is reduced progressively by half (again, 6 dB/octave). Thus, in our example, at the frequency of 70 Hz the amplitude of all components will be attenuated to about 35%, at 140 Hz it will be attenuated to 1.75%, and so on. Again, a line connecting all these points and the maximum can give a good approximation to the response of the filter.

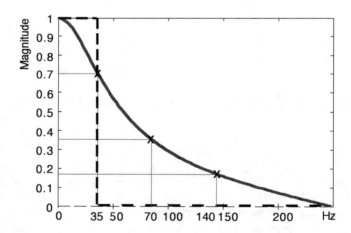

Figure 4.8   Frequency response of an ideal (dashed line) and real (solid line) HFF with cutoff frequency of 35 Hz.

4.4.5   Time Constant

As mentioned earlier, the electronic circuits of filters contain mostly resistors and capacitors, and the latter require a finite amount of time to charge and discharge. The combined effect that resistance and capacitance have on the flow of current when an alternating voltage is applied to the circuit is called the impedance of the filter. The *time constant* of a filter refers to the amount of time necessary for the filter output to respond to a voltage change at its input.

The frequency cutoff and the time constant of a filter are mathematically related. It can be shown that a simple filter, such as the LFF shown in Figure 4.9, consisting of a resistor R and a capacitor C, has a time constant T given by $T = R \times C$, and presents a frequency cutoff f given by $f = \frac{1}{2\pi \times T}$.

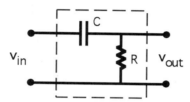

Figure 4.9   Simple LFF filter consisting of a capacitor C and a resistor R.

In many conventional machines using pens and paper, the cutoff frequency of LFFs is reported also in terms of the corresponding time constant, so that it can be used during calibration, which is required at every recording session. Proper function of such a machine can be assessed by measuring the LFF time constants, since it is related to the circuitry of the amplifiers.

From an EEG point of view, the time constant represents the time it takes the EEG pen to fall 63% from its peak amplitude to baseline. In terms of the electronic circuit, this corresponds to the amount of time it takes the capacitor to decay to 37% of its full charge.

The procedure of measuring the time constant of an EEG amplifier is schematically shown in Figure 4.10. In this example, a LFF like the one shown in Figure 4.9 is presented with a pulse at its input. Due to the time needed for the capacitor to go from fully charged to fully discharged, it takes about 1 sec for the output to go from maximum to minimum voltage, and about 0.2 sec for the pen to fall to 37% of its full extent. Thus, in this case, the time constant is 0.2 sec.

Different filter settings, or cutoff frequencies, correspond to different time constants: longer time constants allow lower frequencies to be amplified, while shorter time constants will severely attenuate lower frequencies.

4.4.6   *Notch Filter*

A special category of filters, known as *notch filters,* is useful for removing ideally only one frequency component, such as the 60 Hz interference. In reality, however, these filters attenuate drastically a narrow band of frequencies around that component. As an example, Figure 4.11 shows the frequency response of an ideal (dashed line) and

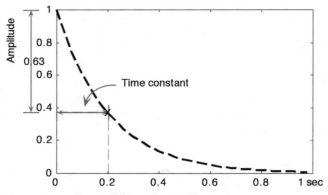

Figure 4.10   Measuring the time constant of an EEG recording system.

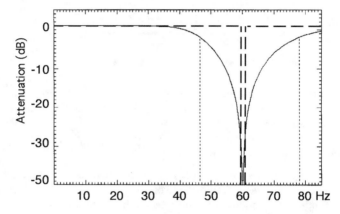

Figure 4.11   Frequency response of an ideal (dashed line) and real (solid line) 60 Hz notch filter.

real (solid line) 60 Hz notch filter. Notice that the cutoff points are around 60 Hz, at 47 and 78 Hz, so that all frequencies in between will be severely attenuated.

Since most useful signals, especially cortical responses, contain components in that frequency range, notch filters should be used only when absolutely necessary, that is, only after *all* other methods of reducing noise (see Chapter 10) have failed.

4.4.7   *Bandwidth*

The frequency range between low and high filter settings will determine the *bandwidth* of the recording system and, thus, the frequency content of the recorded signals. Figure 4.12 depicts the effects of low and high frequency filters on a segment of EEG activity. The original signal is shown in the top of the figure, whereas the middle and bottom parts show the same signal after filtering with an HFF at 5 Hz (all frequencies above 5 Hz removed), or with an LFF at 5 Hz (all frequencies below 5 Hz removed), respectively.

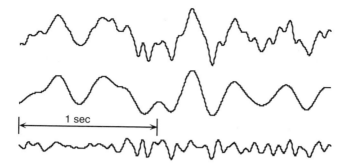

Figure 4.12   Original signal (top) and signal after using a high frequency (middle) and a low frequency (bottom) filter each with a cutoff frequency of 5 Hz.

In general, however, care should be taken in using *any* filter. One should be aware that different neurophysiological signals contain different frequencies; therefore, it is necessary to use different filter settings for each kind of recordings. For example, after stimulation of a peripheral nerve, activity recorded over the spinal cord represents mostly action potentials, whereas activity recorded from the sensory cortex is primarily due to postsynaptic potentials. These two types of activity differ both in duration and frequency content. This implies that the bandwidth of each acquisition amplifier should be adjusted separately to capture the frequency content of the specific signal. Otherwise, a very narrow bandwidth will change the morphology of the useful components by decreasing their amplitude and sharpness. On the other hand, a wider bandwidth will result in noise-contaminated recordings which, in extreme cases, may render the signals unrecognizable. The exact filter settings pertaining to each test are given in Chapters 6 and 7.

4.4.8   Effects of Filtering

Conventional machines use *analog filters* made of resistors and capacitors. Analog filters alter not only the amplitude but also the relative timing of individual waves in a signal. LFF's affect mainly slow waves and make them appear earlier than fast ones, while HFF's attenuate fast components and make them appear later than slow ones [66]. This effect is called *phase shift,* and it is more prominent at frequencies near the cutoff.

Phase shifts are very important when monitoring latency differences among individual components in a waveform, especially in the case of monitoring brainstem auditory evoked responses (BAERs) described in Section 7.5. Changing filter settings, to account for the effects of a new noise source, such as a new piece of equipment brought into the operating room, may also result in a change in the relative timing of individual waves in the waveform, and this may lead to erroneous interpretations.

Modern equipment, on the other hand, relies on *digital filters* or computer programs, that have similar characteristics with analog filters as far as amplitude attenuation is concerned, but they can eliminate phase shifts.

4.4.9   *Analog to Digital Conversion*

Digitization refers to the process of converting the amplitude of an analog signal into a series of numbers, known as time *samples*. The samples are obtained at consecutive discrete points in time, by measuring the amplitude of the continuous signal at a fixed rate.

The procedure of signal sampling is schematically shown in Figure 4.13(a). The solid line shows a small segment of an analog signal, whereas the superimposed dots indicate the values of the corresponding digitized samples.

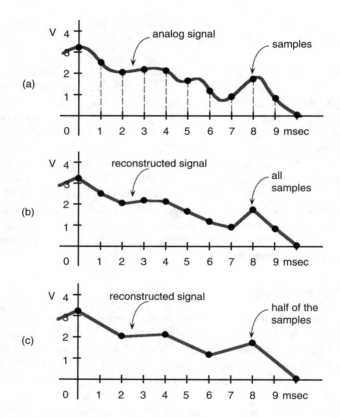

Figure 4.13   (a) Sampling of an analog signal and reconstruction using (b) all samples or (c) every other sample.

The distance between successive samples is determined by the *sampling rate,* which is defined as the number of samples contained in a 1 sec segment of data and simply indicates how often the samples are collected.

The original signal can be reconstructed from the discrete samples, for example, by connecting successive samples with a straight line, but the similarity of the reconstructed signal with the original one will depend on the sampling rate, as Figure 4.13 shows. In part (b) all samples are used to reconstruct the signal, while in part (c) the signal is reconstructed using every other sample. It is obvious that fewer samples give less accurate reconstructions, and most of the signal detail is lost.

Therefore, if the amplitude of the signal to be digitized changes fast, that is if the signal contains high frequencies, a high sampling rate is needed to capture all the signal details. On the other hand, for signals whose amplitude changes slowly, lower sampling rates are adequate for signal reconstruction. For example, to capture the early components of brainstem responses, a sampling on the order of a few thousand samples per second is needed, while to digitize EEG only a few hundred samples per second are required.

4.4.10 Averaging

Averaging is a procedure used to record evoked potentials (EPs), defined in Chapter 2 as the electrical responses of the brain to repeated sensory stimuli (see also Chapter 7). The most common stimuli used in the operating room are auditory tones, for recording BAERs, and electrical pulses, for recording somatosensory EPs.

When recorded on the scalp, EPs are very small compared to the ongoing activity so that individual responses cannot be clearly distinguished. This is because the amount of additional neural signaling due to the stimulus is minute compared to the background signals which correspond to all concurrent functions of the brain, and to other concurrent electrical activity, such as the ECG, muscle activity, and extraneous interference. However, we can use signal averaging to enhance the responses if we make the following assumptions: (1) each stimulus produces some additional neural signaling that is embedded in the seemingly random background activity; (2) all stimuli evoke similar responses that have a constant time relationship to the stimulus; (3) the background noise has a mean value of approximately zero; and (4) the activity resulting from the stimuli is uncorrelated with the ongoing, spontaneous activity.

A portion of activity beginning a few milliseconds before and extending several milliseconds after the presentation of the stimulus is called an *epoch*. The activity specific to the stimulus is usually called the *signal* while all other activity that is unrelated to the stimulus is referred to as *noise*. *Averaging* then serves to extract the signal from the background noise and involves three steps: (1) repeated presentation of a stimulus, (2) recording and addition of each response to the preceding ones, and (3) dividing the sum by the total number of responses.

The averaging procedure is implemented in a computer which can digitize and store each epoch separately. At each time point, corresponding samples across all epochs are added together, sample by sample, and then each sum is divided by number of epochs. The resulting averages are the time samples of the EP.

This process is illustrated in Figure 4.14 where N trials obtained from a single electrode placed at the vertex (C_z) are averaged to produce an EP. Stimuli are delivered at the origin of the time axis.

In multichannel recordings, activity is recorded from several locations on the head simultaneously. Thus, the above procedure is carried out on each channel separately,

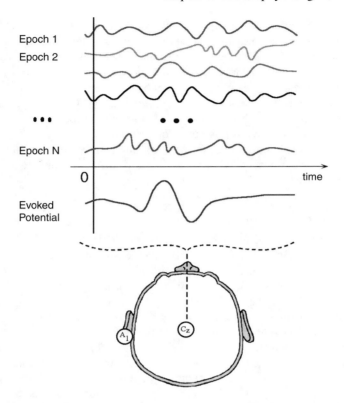

Figure 4.14   Example of averaging N single trials to obtain an evoked potential from a single recording channel.

and yields a separate EP for each recording channel. This case is shown in Figure 4.15, where EPs from M channels are recorded.

The number of trials (N) used to compute the average will affect the signal-to-noise ratio (SNR) of a particular recording: the higher this number, the lower the noise. It can be shown that, under the ideal conditions of zero-mean background noise and constant responses, the SNR improves by a factor equal to the square root of the number of trials used to compute the average ($\sqrt{N}$). Thus, activity time-locked to the stimulus (the EP) is enhanced by the same factor. However, since increased number of trials translates into longer time necessary to obtain the average response, the ability to detect a change during intraoperative recordings decreases as the number of trials increases.

4.5   Data Display

A system should present the results in a way that affords fast interpretation. Typically, real time data collected from several channels simultaneously are plotted on the screen, each with its own time and amplitude scales. Additionally, in a separate area the

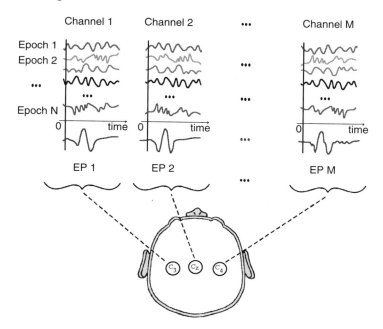

Figure 4.15   In multichannel recordings, a separate evoked potential is obtained from each channel.

system can display current amplitude and latency measurements, along with statistics on the entire data set (from the beginning of the recording session to the current time) in the form of trend plots, spectrograms, etc.

The selection of channels to display should be such that immediate comparisons, for instance between affected and unaffected sides or with baselines usually displayed constantly under the most recent set with a different color, could be easily performed. Displaying of trend plots (successive measurements of the amplitude and/or latency of a specific component in a waveform over time), and of stacks of data (successive plots of an entire waveform over time) should facilitate detection of any significant changes.

4.6   *Data Storage*

Data can be printed on paper during surgery, and they can also be stored on magnetic media, such as hard and/or floppy disks, for off-line review, printing, and permanent storage. Additionally, a network connection may also allow for remote data transmission and monitoring. Typically, all data collected during an operation, along with a report containing the stimulation and recording parameters, the technologist's comments, and the neurophysiologist's interpretation, are included in the patient's record.

4.7   Review Questions

1. What are the two basic characteristics of neurophysiological signals?

2. What does the baseline represent in EEG recordings?

3. What does the spectrum of a signal show?

4. What is the relationship between the duration and the frequency of an EEG wave?

5. What is the frequency of an EEG wave that has a duration of 100 msec?

6. What is the frequency content of a signal obtained by summing two sinusoidals with frequencies 2 Hz and 5 Hz?

7. Explain how the compressed spectral array (CSA) format of a signal is constructed.

8. How is the signal-to-noise ratio defined?

9. What are the names of two common techniques used to reduce noise in a recording?

10. What is the function of a filter?

11. What is the effect of a low frequency filter on an EEG recording?

12. What is the effect of a high frequency filter on an EEG recording?

13. Define the function of a notch filter.

14. What does the frequency response of a filter represent?

15. What is the difference between a linear scale and a logarithmic scale?

16. What does the cutoff frequency represent in a real filter?

17. Draw the frequency response of an ideal low frequency filter with a cutoff at 20 Hz.

18. Draw the frequency response of an ideal high frequency filter with a cutoff at 20 Hz.

19. If the cutoff frequency of a high frequency filter is 50 Hz, what is the attenuation of the filter at 100 Hz?

20. What does the time constant of a filter represent?

21. What is the time constant due to?

22. Is it true that in EEG recordings a longer time constant setting allows lower EEG frequencies to pass?

23. With reference to an EEG machine, what does the time constant represent?

24. Is it true that real notch filters eliminate only one frequency component?

25. What does the bandwidth of a recording system represent?

26. What kind of effects do analog filters have on signals?

27. What is the main advantage of digital filters?

28. What are the assumptions on which signal averaging is based?

29. Why is averaging used in computing evoked potentials?

30. Explain how a single channel EP is computed.

31. Explain how multichannel EPs are computed.

32. When averaging signals, is it true that the signal-to-noise ratio is affected by the number of trials used in the average? If yes, how?

33. What does the sensitivity of an EEG machine represent?

34. Give the formula relating the sensitivity of an EEG machine with the input voltage and the pen deflection.

chapter 5

Anesthesia Management

5.1 Introduction

All neurophysiological signals acquired during surgery, whether reflecting spontaneous or evoked activity, are drastically affected by the anesthesia regime, because
most anesthetic agents affect one or more physiological parameters, such as blood
pressure, blood flow, perfusion, metabolic rate, and neurotransmitter action. In turn,
these parameters determine the function of various neuronal and muscular structures
which are the generators of the signals recorded during monitoring. In order to avoid
erroneous conclusions, interpretation of all neurophysiological recordings should always take into account the effects of changes in anesthesia regime which are very
similar to the changes from surgical intervention.

Certain neuroprotective conditions, such as hypothermia and hypotension, are also
very common; and since they, too, affect neurophysiological signals, they also contribute to the difficulty of correct interpretation of the recordings. Therefore, a quick
overview of the most common drugs and induced conditions is necessary.

However, grouping the various drugs used during neurological, orthopedic, and
neurovascular surgery into different categories is by no means unique, given that
certain anesthetics are frequently used for their nonanesthetic effects, for example, to
reduced blood pressure. Thus, the distinction between anesthetic and nonanesthetic
agents is often unclear. A common approach, however, is to group these drugs into two
major categories, according to the method of administration, namely *inhalational* and
intravenous agents. In the former category, gaseous agents are inhaled and absorbed
through the lungs, whereas in the latter category, anesthetics are injected directly into
the blood stream.

5.2 Components of Anesthesia

General anesthesia consists of several components, including *analgesia* (suppression of response to pain), *sedation* (induction of sleep), *amnesia* (suppression of
recollection of the intraoperative experience), and *muscle relaxation* (suppression of
muscle contraction). It may also include *hypotension* (decreased blood pressure), and
hypothermia (decreased body temperature). Several anesthetic agents will provide

varying degrees of these individual components. However, to avoid the side effects of the more potent drugs which are dose dependent, a commonly used technique is the so-called *balanced anesthesia,* in which several carefully titrated drugs provide each component of general anesthesia.

5.3   Efficacy of Anesthetics

The efficacy of anesthetics is expressed in terms of a MAC, which is defined as "the minimum alveolar concentration (MAC) of anesthetic necessary to prevent movement in 50% of patients in response to surgical stimulation." The actual concentration of drug needed to obtain the effects of one MAC varies among anesthetics. For instance, 1.3% of Isoflurane would be equivalent to 0.7% of Halothane, since they both correspond to one MAC.

5.4   Inhalational Anesthetics

Isoflurane, Halothane, and Enflurane are the most commonly inhalational anesthetics used to provide amnesia, analgesia, sedation, and blood pressure control. Other less common agents include Desflurane and Sevoflurane. Nitrous oxide (N_2O) is typically used as a supplement to these potent, longer-lasting agents, thus allowing their use in smaller concentrations. Except for N_2O which is already a gas, these agents are liquid and they must be converted to gases by vaporization.

5.5   Intravenous Anesthetics

Barbiturates (e.g., Thiopental, and Methohexital) are commonly used for induction and rarely for maintenance of anesthesia, since in high doses they delay awakening and prolong the time to extubation.

Opiates (e.g., morphine and synthetic narcotics, such as Fentanyl, Alfentanil, and Sufentanil) can induce anesthesia while maintaining hemodynamic stability. Narcotics constitute an essential component of balanced anesthesia because they provide profound analgesia.

Benzodiazepines (e.g., Diazepam and Midazolam) are typically used before induction of anesthesia.

Propofol is a commonly used anesthetic primarily because of its very short duration of action. It can be used for both induction and maintenance of anesthesia.

Etomidate can also be used for both induction and maintenance, and it is especially useful for providing hemodynamic stability.

Ketamine can be used for induction of anesthesia and can maintain hemodynamic stability. However, its use is very rare because of possible postoperative hallucinations.

5.6   Neuroprotective Agents

Mannitol is used during neurosurgery to reduce brain swelling in patients with cerebral edema. It has been shown to increase cerebral blood flow in the ischemic brain, and to decrease blood viscosity. However, its ability to preserve electrical activity in the brain or the spinal cord has yet to be demonstrated.

Barbiturates have been suggested as neuroprotective agents in cerebral ischemia by decreasing the cerebral metabolic rate. This effect is maximal when EEG burst suppression is attained.

Corticosteroids, such as Dexamethasone and Methylprednisolone, are thought to have neuroprotective effects in cerebral edema resulting from ischemia. High doses of steroids have been shown to have beneficial effects in spinal cord injury if administered within the first 8 hours from injury. Because of side effects, however, their use still remains controversial in certain cases.

5.7   Protective Induced Conditions

5.7.1   Muscle Relaxation

Muscle relaxation is typically used in neurological and orthopedic surgery to prevent patient movement which, in certain cases, might have devastating results. It is also used to facilitate tissue retraction. Depending on the type and dose of the agent, induced paralysis may last from a few minutes to an hour. Muscle relaxants are typically administered intravenously.

With reference to their speed of action these agents are divided into two categories: (1) Fast-acting relaxants, such as Succinylcholine, induce paralysis in about 30 sec and their effects last for approximately 4 min. They are typically used during induction to control the airways, and (2) slow-acting relaxants, such as Vecuronium, Pancuronium, and Atracurium, need about 3 min to induce paralysis, but their effects may last for up to one hour.

Depth of muscle relaxation is monitored by delivering a series of four electrical pulses, usually to the median or facial nerve, and measuring the resulting twitches from the patient. Zero twitches indicates complete paralysis, whereas four twitches indicate practically no paralysis.

5.7.2   Other Conditions

Hypotension, or reduced blood pressure, is commonly used as a way to reduce blood loss. It can be induced in several ways: by increasing the concentration of inhalational anesthetics, such as Isoflurane; through a bolus injection of an anesthetic, like Propofol or Thiopental; or more commonly, by using a vasoactive agent, such as Nitroprusside or Nitroglycerin.

Hypothermia, or decreased body temperature, has been shown to provide protective benefits against cerebral and spinal injuries, cerebral hemorrhage, and even cardiac arrest. Mild hypothermia (around 33^oC) is currently used for its protective effects against cerebral ischemia.

Hyperventilation, or increased respiration, is used intraoperatively to reduce carbon dioxide (CO_2), and the total volume of the brain by decreasing its blood volume. The benefit from this is better exposure and less tissue retraction which reduce the risk of injury.

Hypervolemia, or expansion of the blood volume, has been shown to provide protective benefits against cerebral ischemia.

5.8   Effects on Neurophysiological Signals

The effects of most anesthetic agents on spontaneous neurophysiological activity are dose dependent. Practically all anesthetics in small doses initially increase the frequency content of the EEG and then, at higher doses, they introduce some high-amplitude, low-frequency waves.

Anesthetics affect somatosensory evoked potentials in a similar way, by decreasing the amplitude and increasing the latency mostly of the cortical components, again in a dose-dependent fashion. Probably the only two exceptions to this rule are Etomidate and Ketamine, which can actually increase the amplitude of cortical responses by up to 600% [43].

In general, inhalational agents have more dramatic effects than injectable anesthetics, especially in concentrations higher than 0.5 MAC. On the other hand, a *bolus injection,* that is, a one-shot, large dose of an anesthetic may completely obliterate cortical responses for about 15 min after the injection. So, whenever possible, the preferred form of administration would be intravenous drip infusion which delivers drugs more slowly over a longer period of time, at a constant rate.

The effects of blood pressure changes on evoked potentials are not significant if the mean arterial pressure is not reduced below 60 mmHg, and if it is controlled through vasoactive agents (e.g., Nitroprusside) rather than inhalational anesthetics (e.g., Isoflurane).

Similarly, mild hypothermia does not have significant effects on brain activity, and it may only increase slightly the latency of components. However, at lower body temperatures the effects are more dramatic (see Section 6.2.6).

The exact effects that these agents and conditions have on various neurophysiological recordings are described in detail in Chapters 6 and 7.

5.9   Review Questions

1. Explain how neurophysiological signals are affected by anesthetic agents.

2. What are the two main categories of anesthetic agents?

3. Describe the various components of anesthesia.

4. What does the term "balanced anesthesia" mean?

5. How is the efficacy of anesthetics measured?

6. What are the names of a few very common inhalational anesthetics?

7. What is the effect of barbiturates on the EEG and on EPs?

8. What is the effect of narcotics on EPs?

9. Do muscle relaxants affect EPs?

10. What is the effect of inhalational agents on EPs?

11. Does nitrous oxide affect EPs? If yes, how?

12. What is the effect of Propofol on EPs?

13. Which drug can be used to enhance the amplitude of cortical EPs?

14. What are the names of some common neuroprotective agents?

15. What protective induced conditions are typically used in neurosurgical procedures?

16. Describe the typical overall effects that anesthetic agents have on neurophysiological signals as the dose increases.

chapter 6

Spontaneous Activity

6.1 Introduction

Several structures in the body are generators of spontaneous bioelectrical activity that can be easily recorded externally. All these generators are part of the nervous or the muscular system. For instance, neurons in the brain produce what is usually recorded on the scalp as the electroencephalogram (EEG), while contracting muscles give rise to the signals typically captured in an electromyogram (EMG).

Intraoperative monitoring procedures rely on the fact that the various patterns of surface-recorded bioelectrical signals provide information on the structural and functional integrity of the underlying generators, and more generally on the neural pathways to which these generators belong.

One way to obtain this information is by observing *directly* the activity of neuronal structures. For instance, in the case of cortical *ischemia,* a condition associated with a drastic decrease in blood supply to the cerebral cortex, EEG monitoring provides a direct and sensitive way to detect and quantify any changes in brain activity.

However, information can also be obtained *indirectly,* given the intimate interconnection between the muscular and the nervous systems. Indeed, muscles are always activated by signals coming from a motor nerve. Thus, observing patterns of muscular activity can provide information about the integrity of the nerves innervating that muscle. This is a very common approach with operations that may put at risk various cranial nerves or spinal nerve roots which often are not easily accessible to obtain direct recordings.

In this chapter, we focus on EEG and EMG recordings not as diagnostic tools, but as neuroprotective intraoperative monitoring procedures. We give specific details regarding the information these signals can provide, the appropriate electrode types and placement locations, as well as typical acquisition parameters and factors that affect the recorded activity. Finally, we provide some suggestions for real-time interpretation of the intraoperative results.

6.2   Electroencephalogram

6.2.1   Generation

The EEG provides a quantitative measure for the spontaneous electrical activity of the brain, that can be obtained by surface electrodes placed on the scalp. As explained in Section 2.4.3, the EEG is generated by vast numbers of pyramidal cells [65] in the cerebral cortex, which is organized in layers of tissue. A schematic diagram of this is shown in Figure 2.7.

Because of this particular arrangement, electrical signals generated in the cortex must cross several layers of tissue before reaching the recording electrodes on the scalp, as is schematically shown in Figure 6.1. All these tissues, namely the meninges, the cerebrospinal fluid, and the skull, have a different conductivity, thus they will affect the EEG signal in a different fashion. Furthermore, different brain structures are interlinked through an intricate network of connections spanning both hemispheres [29]. All these factors add to the reduced spatial resolution of the EEG, which can sometimes result in misleading indications as to the exact site of a compromised cortical area [70].

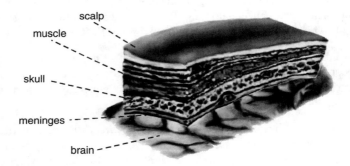

Figure 6.1   Several layers of tissues intervene between the brain, where the EEG signal is generated, and the scalp, the surface recording sites.

6.2.2   Use

Clinically, the EEG has been used extensively as a noninvasive tool in the diagnosis and assessment of many disease states of the brain, including epilepsy, coma, tumors, and stroke. It has also been used in the definition and study of anesthesia and of sleep stages.

Intraoperatively, however, the EEG is used exclusively for monitoring cerebral function. The normal function of neurons depends on proper supply of oxygen and glucose, both of which are provided by the cerebral circulation. Approximately 40% of the total metabolic rate for oxygen in the brain is used to keep neurons alive, that is, to sustain the membrane structure and the basic metabolic state in cells, whereas the remaining 60% is used for neurophysiological functions [70].

A decrease in blood supply diminishes oxygen availability and poses a direct threat to neurons, which cannot survive for more than 3–5 min without proper oxygenation [59]. Under ischemia conditions, neurons will preserve *structure* rather than *function*. That is, in an effort to preserve energy and stay alive, they will cease neurophysiological function, and as result electrophysiological recordings will be the first to be affected [70]. Therefore, continuous monitoring of the EEG activity can provide an early warning of an imminent catastrophe.

In general, when there is a reduction in blood supply to the brain, the EEG deteriorates. The earliest warning is a change in the EEG frequency content. More specifically, it is characterized by a decrease or even loss of high-frequency components which is accompanied by an increase in high-amplitude slower components [59]. More severe ischemia results in EEG fragmentation, also known as *burst suppression.* In that case, periods of electrical silence alternate with periods of activity, eventually leading to a complete electrical silence or "flat EEG." However, the sequence of changes may be reversed without brain damage, if an adequate oxygen supply is restored early enough [70].

Certain surgical procedures involve temporary arrest of blood flow to specific areas of the brain, usually by clamping an artery. Typically, following clamping, collateral circulation provides for proper oxygenation of the neurons in the areas supplied by the occluded vessel.

However, a sudden drop in blood flow, for example, due to rapture of the occluded vessel or to unintentional occlusion of a different near by artery, may cause an ischemic or a hemorrhagic stroke. Depending on the severity of the event and the location of the affected area of the brain, the patient may develop several deficits, ranging from temporary unilateral weakness to permanent total paralysis. In these kinds of surgery, continuous monitoring before, during, and after arresting the blood flow provides a reliable index of blood perfusion in the brain areas that are involved in surgery.

Thus, procedures such as carotid endarterectomy (Section 9.5), aneurysm clipping, or repair of an arteriovenous malformation (AVM, Section 9.3), and balloon angioplasty (Section 9.6) are excellent candidates for EEG monitoring. These procedures will be described in more detail in their respective sections of the book.

6.2.3   *EEG Features*

Three basic features of the EEG are most relevant in the operating room: *amplitude, frequency,* and bilateral *symmetry* over homotopic sites on the two hemispheres.

The *amplitude* of the EEG usually varies from 10 to 100 μV, and it can be roughly separated into low, medium, or high if activity has a value of less than 20 μV, between 20 and 50 μV, or more than 50 μV, respectively.

The *frequency* range between 0.1 and 30 Hz contains most of the clinically important EEG activity. This range has been traditionally divided into four bands: *delta,* between 0.1–4 Hz; *theta,* between 4–8 Hz; *alpha,* between 8–13 Hz; and *beta,* between 13–30 Hz [20]. Interestingly, as the frequency increases, the amplitude of the EEG decreases, and vice versa.

An awake but relaxed subject shows activity mainly in the alpha range that changes into a mixture of alpha and beta during mental activity. Alpha frequencies are more prominent in the occipital areas, whereas beta frequencies are mostly seen in frontal regions. During sleep, a combination of theta and slow delta activity dominates the EEG patterns. Under anesthesia, however, the normal EEG contains a mixture of slow and fast frequencies uniformly distributed on the entire head.

Regardless of the mental stage of a subject, whether he or she is awake, asleep, or under anesthesia, normal EEG activity is symmetrical over the two hemispheres, as far as morphology, amplitude, and frequency content are concerned.

The amplitude, frequency content, and symmetry of the EEG can be obtained on-line through visual inspection of the traces, or from power spectrum plots. In particular, as explained in Section 4.3.3, plotting the activity of a specific channel in *compressed spectral array* (CSA) format, can clearly visualize the evolution in time of the dominant EEG frequencies from that channel.

6.2.4   Recording Procedure

For proper intraoperative monitoring, it is not necessary—and most likely not possible, due to surgical field constraints—to use the large number of channels typically employed in diagnostic EEG. Instead, it is sufficient to use an anteroposterior bipolar montage with *at least* three electrodes placed symmetrically on each side of the head: one frontal, one centroparietal, and one occipital. An example of such an arrangement is shown in Figure 6.2, where a total of four EEG channels according to the 10–20 International System are available, namely F_7–C_3', C_3'–O_1, F_8–C_4', and C_4'–O_2, with a ground electrode on the forehead, at F_{pz}. The primed electrodes C_3' and C_4' are placed about 2 cm posteriorly to C_3 and C_4, respectively.

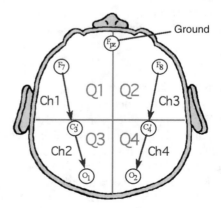

Figure 6.2   Intraoperative EEG recording protocol using four channels that form four quadrants for monitoring brain activity.

Notice the four quadrants, Q_1 to Q_4 formed by this montage, which allows for continuous comparison of the activity on the hemisphere involved with surgery with the activity on the homotopic unaffected side. Thus, it is possible to detect changes in the anterior, posterior, left, or right quadrant, independently. For instance, in case of ischemia during a carotid endarterectomy procedure (Section 9.5), the various brain regions would be affected unequally, and this asymmetry would also be reflected on the signals recorded from these regions.

It should be noted, however, that the suggested minimal montage provides satisfactory monitoring if, in addition to EEG, other tests, such as somatosensory evoked potentials (see Section 7.3.5), are being administered simultaneously. Otherwise, a minimum of sixteen channels of EEG covering the parasagittal and temporal regions is recommended [39].

The preferred type of recording electrodes are hypodermic sterile needles because, as explained in Section 3.5, they are easy to use and they maintain a stable impedance of a long period of time. Again, the desired electrode impedance is less than 2 kΩ.

The segment of EEG data displayed on the screen is called the *time base*. At any given time it should be long enough to allow for proper recognition of patterns of brain activity and detection of possible changes. Thus, depending on the size of the computer monitor, each screen should contain between 5–10 sec of activity. A typical display may look like the example in Figure 6.3, which was recorded during a carotid endarterectomy procedure. Notice that homotopic sites show symmetrical activity.

Filter settings should be such that all clinically useful frequencies are preserved, while extraneous noise is rejected. Therefore, the low- and high-pass filters should be set at 1 and 30 Hz, respectively. Table 6.1 summarizes the parameter settings for the minimum montage recommended for intraoperative EEG monitoring.

Table 6.1 Parameter Settings Recommended for Intraoperative EEG Monitoring

Hemisphere	Channels	Bandwidth	Time Base
Left	F_7–C_3'		
	C_3'–O1	1–30 Hz	5–10 sec
Right	F_8–C_4'		
	C_4'–O2		

6.2.5 Effects of Anesthetic Agents

The effects of drugs on arterial blood flow, intracranial pressure, and cerebral perfusion pressure will result in changes of the EEG patterns that are a function of depth of anesthesia.

Normally, light anesthesia results in a widespread EEG activity that contains low-amplitude, high-frequency waves mixed with high-amplitude, low-frequency

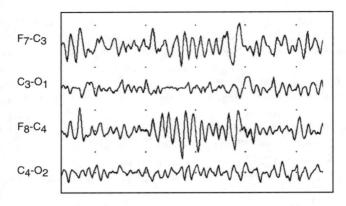

Figure 6.3   Example of intraoperative EEG recording. (Notice the symmetry of activity on homotopic recording channels.)

ones [39, 43, 70]. This pattern is uniform over the entire head and common to most anesthetized patients under typical depths of anesthesia.

At deeper anesthesia stages, waves of higher amplitude and lower frequency appear, while short periods of burst suppression may also occur occasionally. If anesthesia depth progresses further, bursts of activity are followed by longer periods of suppression, until total EEG silence (also known as *isoelectricity*) is reached [39, 43]. At such high concentrations, certain anesthetics may produce seizure-like activity, or spikes, rather than isoelectricity.

The effect of depth of anesthesia on the EEG is shown in the example of Figure 6.4. Initially, continuous activity is observed, as Figure 6.4(a) shows, and then, at deeper stages, bursts of activity are followed by segments of activity suppression, as seen in Figure 6.4(b).

The specific action of several anesthetic agents on the EEG has been described in detail elsewhere [21, 39, 43, 70]. The effects of some of the most commonly used drugs and induced neuroprotective conditions are outlined next, and they are also summarized in Table 6.2.

Inhalation Anesthetics

For gaseous agents, there is an empirically determined reference value of anesthetic called a MAC (minimum anesthetic concentration), which is defined as the alveolar concentration necessary to prevent movement in 50% of subjects in response to surgical incision [19].

Nitrous oxide (N_2O) at 50% concentration, which is equivalent to 0.6 MAC, reduces alpha and introduces short burst of beta activity. At 80% concentration all fast activity disappears and the EEG contains only theta activity [20].

Isoflurane, Halothane, and *Enflurane* are the most common inhalational anesthetics. All three agents in small concentrations, approximately 0.6 MAC [43], increase the frequency and reduce the amplitude of the EEG, but at higher concentrations (anesthetic doses), they produce a dose-dependent slowing [21]. Increased doses

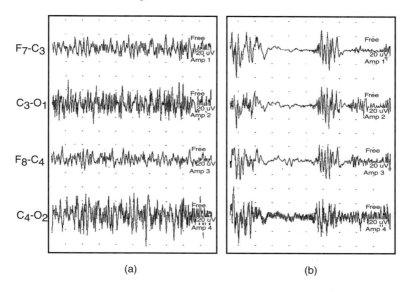

(a)   (b)

Figure 6.4 Example showing the effects of anesthesia depth on the EEG. (a) At typical depths, a generalized pattern of activity is seen on the entire head, whereas (b) at deeper stages, bursts of activity are followed by burst suppression.

result, in the case of Isoflurane, in burst suppression and, in the case of Enflurane, in epileptic-like bursts [39] followed by isoelectricity. The typical EEG frequencies observed at 1 MAC concentration when each agent is administered alone are as follows: Halothane (0.75%), activity between 11–16 Hz; Enflurane (1.7%), activity between 4-8 Hz; and Isoflurane (1.3%), activity between 15–16 Hz. If N_2O is given together with these agents, slowing occurs at lower concentrations.

Intravenous Agents

Propofol in sedative concentrations produces a dramatic increase in beta, followed by an increase in alpha and beta activity. At higher concentration, an increase in delta activity, with almost no change in theta band activity is observed, and ultimately burst suppression is produced [70]. If N_2O is given together with Propofol, the maximum activity observed is mainly in the alpha band [20].

Benzodiazepines, such as Diazepam and Midazolam, produce EEG changes similar to Propofol.

Barbiturates, such as Thiopental and Methohexital, have dose-dependent effects on the EEG that start with the production of fast activity (15–30 Hz). This is followed by the appearance of slower waves (5–12 Hz) which are superimposed on the fast activity in spindles. Increased concentrations result in high-amplitude slower waves (1–3 Hz). Increased doses result in burst suppression which, at higher doses, is followed by electrocortical silence [43].

Etomidate, a nonbarbiturate, produces EEG changes similar to barbiturates.

Opiates, such as Morphine, and synthetic narcotics, such as Fentanyl, Alfentanil,

Table 6.2   Effects of Anesthetic Agents on EEG Amplitude and
Frequency at Typical Doses

Agent	Amplitude	Frequency
Nitrous Oxide (N_2O)	⇓	⇑
Inhalational Anesthetics Isoflurane, Halothane, Enflurane, Desflurane	⇓	⇑
Propofol	⇓	⇑
Barbiturates Thiopental, Methohexital	⇓	⇑
Etomidate	⇓	⇑
Opiates Morphine, Fentanyl, Alfentanil, Sufentanil	↑	⇓
Benzodiazepines Diazepam, Midazolam	⇓	⇑
Muscle Relaxants Saccinycholine, Pancuronium, Vecuronium	—	—
Hypotensive Agents Nitroprusside, Nitroglycerin	⇓	⇓

Note: ↑ or ↓: modest change; ⇑ or ⇓: significant change; —: no change.

and Sufentanil, cause a dose-dependent EEG slowing, with a maximum effect resulting in activity in the delta band [70].

6.2.6   Effects of Induced Neuroprotective Conditions

Hypothermia, or body temperature of less than 35°C, progressively reduces the frequency of the EEG in a temperature-dependent fashion. This is followed by an
amplitude reduction, while intermittent burst suppression starts at about 26°C [43].
Finally, total suppression is seen in profound hypothermia to less than 20°C [59].

Hypotension, or reduced blood pressure, results in EEG slowing when cerebral
perfusion pressure drops below 50 mmHg [20]. Thus, in the intact brain, the EEG
does not change significantly even when arterial blood pressure is lowered to about
50% of its initial value [3]. However, certain vasoactive agents, such as Nitroprusside
and Nitroglycerin, which are used to reduce arterial blood pressure, may also reduce
cerebral perfusion pressure [42] which, in turn, results in EEG slowing.

Hypercarbia, or increased levels of carbon dioxide (CO_2) that may result, for
example, from hypoventilation, decreases cerebral perfusion pressure and thus results

in EEG slowing [3]. CO_2 at 30% concentration results in intermittent epileptiform discharges [20].

6.2.7   *Effects of Age*

Low-amplitude, nonrhythmic, poorly defined, random-frequency waves in the delta, theta, and alpha ranges are normally seen in newborn infants. As age progresses, the EEG shows rhythmic patterns and, by the age of 1 year, activity in the theta range is detected. By the age of 8 years, alpha activity within the adult frequency range is clearly seen. The elderly (more than 80 years of age) show intermittent temporal slowing in the EEG [34].

6.2.8   *EEG Intraoperative Interpretation*

Typically, upon induction of anesthesia, the EEG shows onset of widespread slowing (theta and high delta activity) and, at the same time, built-up of fast (beta) activity. Thus, the background EEG of a normal subject under typical levels of anesthesia contains a mixture of slow and fast frequencies. This pattern is uniform over the entire head and, in the absence of any additional pharmacological or surgical manipulation, it should remain stable throughout the operation.

Any changes in the normal pattern during surgery can be due to either ischemia, resulting from surgical maneuvering, such as, for instance, from the placement of an artery clamp, or to perisurgical factors, which include alterations in depth of anesthesia and body temperature, or administration of a bolus injection of drugs.

The effects on EEG from ischemia depend on the site of insult and are manifested commonly as follows: *ischemia of the cerebral cortex* typically results in a sudden, localized reduction or total loss of high frequency waves, followed by the appearance of high-amplitude slow waves in the delta band. Long intervals of cortical ischemia will produce a further decrease in both the amplitude and frequency of the EEG, until isoelectricity (EEG silence) is reached [20]. Often, however, *ischemia of the internal capsule* or the *thalamus* produces undetectable changes in the EEG. *Brainstem ischemia,* on the other hand, appears as a widespread amplitude decrease accompanied by generalized slowing [20].

Unfortunately, several anesthetic agents may have similar effects on the EEG. In general, however, EEG changes due to ischemia are abrupt and localized. That is, they occur within seconds and affect mostly only one hemisphere. On the other hand, changes from perisurgical factors are relatively slow and generalized, that is, they happen over the course of several minutes and affect both hemispheres equally and simultaneously.

Therefore, successful differentiation of EEG changes due to ischemia from changes due to perisurgical factors can be achieved by correlating the observed EEG changes with surgical maneuvers, anesthesia regime, blood pressure, oxygen level, heart rate, body temperature, and administration of drugs.

6.3   Electromyogram

6.3.1   Generation

A record of the electrical activity of a muscle is called an electromyogram (EMG). As explained in Section 2.4.5, this activity is due to temporal and spatial summation of postsynaptic muscle action potentials generated on several muscle fibers after a stimulus from a motor neuron has reached the muscle [72].

The response of individual fibers is of the *all-or-none* type. That is, each fiber is either completely stretched or not stretched at all. However, the response of the whole muscle depends on the number of fibers excited.

Stronger muscle contraction can be obtained by either increasing the number of fibers responding to stimulation or by increasing the frequency of contractions of each fiber. Successive stimuli from a motor neuron have an additive effect if they are applied fast enough, so that the second stimulus arrives before the muscle has relaxed completely [72]. The frequency of stimulation can be increased progressively until a maximum contraction, known as *tetanus,* is reached. If the total time of contraction is prolonged, the muscle fatigues because its biochemical energy sources are depleted.

6.3.2   Use

Intraoperatively, spontaneous EMG monitoring is used to protect cranial nerves and spinal nerve roots from injury, due to excessive retraction, or unintended dissection. Monitoring the muscles innervated by these nerves for the presence of any kind of activity provides information regarding the integrity of the nerves themselves. Indeed, the presence of muscle activity would indicate that some sort of irritation of the nerve has taken place, and also that the pathway to the muscle is intact.

Several surgical procedures require manipulations that can cause mechanical, thermal, or electrical irritation of nerves and nerve roots. For example, during posterior fossa surgery several adjacent cranial nerves are at risk for damage [47, 75]. Similarly, during spine surgery for stenosis [56], pedicle screw placement [10], or during selective rhizotomy for relief of spasticity [67], spinal nerve roots are at a great risk. Thus, all these procedures are good candidates for EMG monitoring. However, it should be noted that only nerves with a motor division can be monitored through EMG, thus cranial nerves I (Olfactory), II (Optic), and VIII (Vestibulocochlear) are excluded.

Compared to other intraoperative tests for monitoring spinal roots, such as SEP (Section 7.3) and DSEP (Section 7.4), spontaneous EMG has the advantage of being root-specific. Moreover, since there is no need for averaging, it can provide real time feedback.

6.3.3   EMG Features

Contrary to clinical EMG, where the goal is to detect activity in a specific section of a muscle, intraoperative EMG monitoring aims at detecting activity that may occur in *any* section of a muscle or *any* adjacent muscles. Furthermore, intraoperative EMG interpretation is based primarily on the presence or absence of muscle activity and partially on the specific pattern [5]. This implies that the exact EMG amplitude or latency are not as important. For this reason, the recording electrodes should have a large exposed surface in order to sample as wide an area of the muscle as possible.

6.3.4 Recording Procedure

When monitoring cranial nerves, recordings are mostly monopolar. That is, the active electrodes are placed in the muscles innervated by the nerve at risk, while the reference electrode is placed on an indifferent site, such as the cheek contralateral to the side of surgery. The muscles typically used for monitoring cranial nerves [47] are listed in Table 6.3, while the anatomical location of these muscles are graphically depicted in Figures 6.5 to 6.9. Cranial nerve XI can be monitored from the trapezius muscle which is shown in Figure 6.10(a). It cannot be emphasized enough that *extreme* care is needed when placing needle electrodes in the face, especially in muscles around the eyes, a procedure that should be attempted *only* by specially trained personnel.

Table 6.3 Muscles Typically Used for Monitoring the Integrity of Cranial Nerves

Cranial Nerve	Nerve Name	Muscle Monitored
III	Oculomotor	Inferior Rectus
IV	Trochlear	Superior Oblique
V	Trigeminal	Masseter
VI	Abducens	Lateral Rectus
VII	Facial	Orbicularis Oris and Oculi
IX	Glossopharyngeal	Stylopharyngeus
X	Vagus	Cricothyroid
XI	Spinal Accessory	Trapezius
XII	Hypoglossal	Tongue

In the case of monitoring spinal roots, both the ipsilateral and the contralateral muscles are monitored simultaneously, because of anatomical variations in innervation and reflex events in the spinal cord. Thus, recordings are bipolar. That is, the active and the reference electrodes are placed a few centimeters apart, both over the motor point of a muscle. Although each muscle is thought to be supplied primarily from one motor root, the same root may innervate more than one muscle; thus responses may be detected on several muscles simultaneously. For the same reason, the choice of which particular muscle to monitor is based not only on the rootlet at risk, but also on the easiness of muscle identification and electrode insertion. There exist excellent anatomical guides [58] that describe all the necessary steps for identifying muscles properly and for inserting needles correctly.

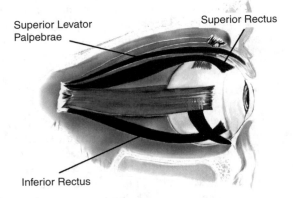

Figure 6.5   Eye muscles used to monitor cranial nerve III.

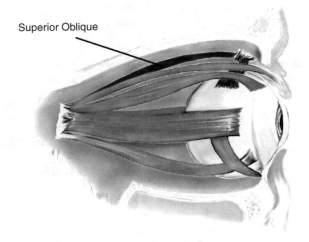

Figure 6.6   Eye muscles used to monitor cranial nerve IV.

Table 6.4 summarizes the muscles used for monitoring cervical, lumbar, and sacral nerve roots. These muscles have been selected because they are large and easy to identify. Figures 6.10 to 6.15 depict graphically how to identify the correct location for placing the stimulating electrodes on arm, hip, and leg muscles.

More specifically, as Figure 6.10 shows, the insertion point on the *upper trapezius* is at the angle of the neck and shoulder, while on the *anterior deltoid* is found about three finger breadths below the anterior *acromion* (the edge of the shoulder). Similarly, the insertion point on the *biceps brachii,* shown in Figure 6.11(a), is at the mid point on the anterior part of the arm, and exactly behind it is the point corresponding to the long head of the *triceps* as shown in Figure 6.11(b). In the *flexor carpi ulnaris* muscle the insertion point is found at the junction of the upper and middle thirds of the forearm, as shown in Figure 6.11(c).

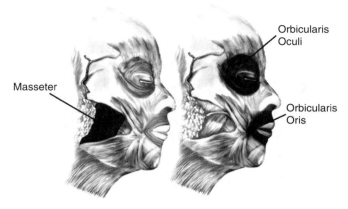

Figure 6.7   Face muscles used to monitor cranial nerve V and VII.

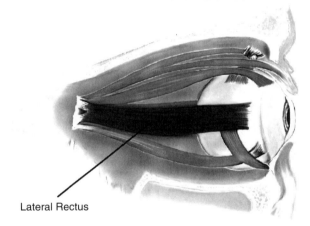

Figure 6.8   Eye muscles used to monitor cranial nerve VI.

The insertion point on the *sartorius* muscle is more difficult to identify but, as Figure 6.12(a) shows, it can be found on the anterior part of the hip about four finger breadths along the line connecting the anterior superior iliac spine (ASIS) and the medial epicondyle (ME) at the knee. On the other hand, the insertion point on the much larger *rectus femoris* muscle is very easy to identify at about half the distance between ASIS and the patella at the knee, indicated as point P in Figure 6.12(b).

On the *tibialis anterior* muscle, shown in Figure 6.13, the insertion point is found about four finger breadths below the lower edge of the knee and about one finger breadth lateral to the tibial crest.

Figure 6.14(a) shows that the insertion point on the long head of the *biceps femoris* muscle is found approximately half the distance between the popliteal crease of the calf and the buttocks. Similarly, the insertion point on the (medial or lateral head of the) *gastrocnemius* muscle is found about one hand breadth below the popliteal crease, as shown in Figure 6.14(b).

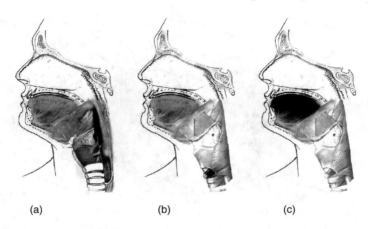

(a)   (b)   (c)

Figure 6.9   Muscles used to monitor cranial nerve, (a) stylophoryngeous, (b) cricothyroid, and (c) tongue.

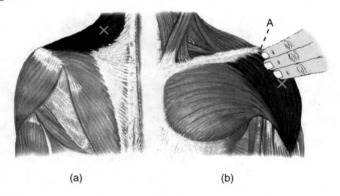

(a)   (b)

Figure 6.10   Identification of the electrode insertion point (x) on the (a) upper trapezius and (b) deltoid muscles.

Finally, for the external *anal sphincter,* shown in Figure 6.14, the electrode should be inserted about two finger breadths laterally from the edge of the rectum. Again, extreme care should be taken to avoid piercing the rectal mucosa.

Typical parameters for recording EMG are as follows: low and high frequency filters set at 5 Hz and 5 kHz, respectively; analysis time set at 50 msec; and sensitivity set at a relatively low value between 50 and 100 mV. These values are summarized in Table 6.5.

6.3.5   Affecting Factors

The most important factor affecting EMG monitoring is the level of muscle relaxation, or the level of pharmacologically induced paralysis, as described in Section 5.7.1. The latter is typically determined by delivering a train of four electrical stimuli, with an

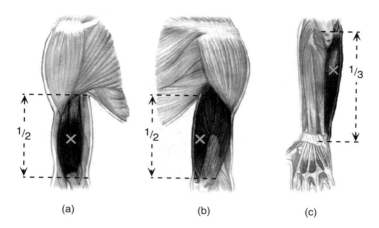

Figure 6.11   Identification of the electrode insertion point (x) on the (a) biceps brachii, (b) long head of the triceps, and (c) flexor carpi ulnaris muscles.

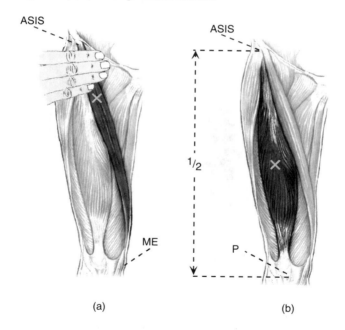

Figure 6.12   Identification of the electrode insertion point (x) on the (a) sartorius and (b) rectus femoris muscles, using as anatomical references the anterior superior iliac spine (ASIS), the medial epicondyle (ME), and the patella (P).

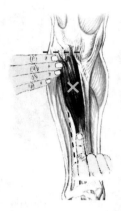

Figure 6.13   Identification of the electrode insertion point (x) on the tibialis anterior muscle.

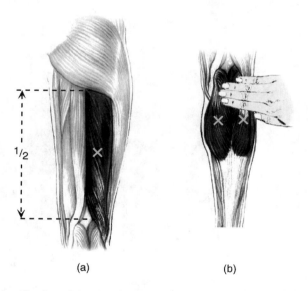

Figure 6.14   Identification of the electrode insertion point (x) on the (a) biceps femoris and (b) the medial (left) or lateral (right) head of the gastrocnemius muscle.

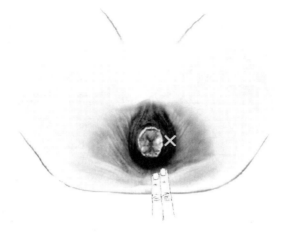

Figure 6.15   Identification of the electrode insertion point (x) on the external anal sphincter muscle.

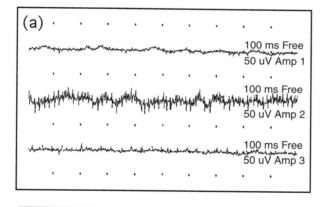

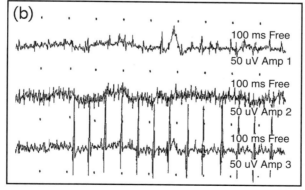

Figure 6.16   Example of EMG activity. (a) Baseline recordings. Note the low amplitude background activity on channel #2. (b) High amplitude spikes are present on channel #3 indicating irritation of the nerve corresponding to that channel.

Table 6.4   Muscles Typically Used for Monitoring the Integrity of Cervical, Lumbar, and Sacral Nerve Roots

Area	Nerve Root	Muscle Monitored
	C_3	Trapezius
	C_4	Trapezius
Cervical	C_5	Deltoid
	C_6	Biceps
	C_7	Triceps
	C_8	Flexor carpi ulnaris
	L_1	Sartorius, iliopsoas
	L_2	Rectus femoris, vastus lateralis
Lumbar	L_3	Rectus femoris, vastus lateralis
	L_4	Tibialis anterior, rectus femoris
	L_5	Tibialis anterior, biceps femoris
	S_1	Biceps femoris
Sacral	S_2	Gastrocnemius, biceps femoris
	S_3	Anal sphincter
	S_4	Anal sphincter

Table 6.5   Parameter Settings Recommended for Intraoperative EMG Monitoring

Bandwidth	Sensitivity	Time Base
5 Hz–5 kHz	50–100 mV	50 msec

intensity of about 25 mA, to the ulnar or the facial nerve and observing the number of muscle contractions elicited. If a patient is *reversed*, or not relaxed at all, there will be four muscle contractions; otherwise, if the patient is completely relaxed, there will be no muscle contractions at all. For monitoring purposes, anesthesia regime must be such that the patient remains minimally relaxed, showing at least three twitches out of a train of four stimuli.

6.3.6   EMG Intraoperative Interpretation

EMG monitoring is greatly facilitated by making the EMG signal audible, so that both the neurophysiologist and the surgeon can hear it [47]. Since the EMG has a characteristic sound reminiscent of "popping popcorn," it is relatively easy to detect various patterns of activity and, also, discriminate real EMG from noise.

The example in Figure 6.16(a) shows baseline EMG activity recorded from three different cranial nerves, with channel #2 having some low amplitude background activity. In Figure 6.16(b) the high amplitude spikes present on channel #3, while the other two channels remain silent, are indicative of real muscle activity, suggesting some irritation of the nerve corresponding to the muscle monitored on channel #3.

Interpretation criteria for possible nerve injury include the following: (1) sustained firing of a high frequency train lasting for tens of seconds, (2) several large bursts of activity of complex morphology, or (3) sudden bursts of high amplitude spikes followed by complete silence [5, 47].

On the contrary, small background activity or a few transient spikes are usually not suggestive of injury. Furthermore, erratic activity that appears simultaneously on all recording channels most likely represents noise.

6.4   *Review Questions*

1. What kinds of spontaneous activity are typically recorded in the operating room?

2. Is it true that information regarding the functional integrity of neuronal structures can be obtained both directly and indirectly? Explain.

3. What are the generators of the EEG signal?

4. What is the clinical use of the EEG?

5. What is the intraoperative use of the EEG?

6. Explain how the EEG can provide an early warning of an ischemic attack in the brain.

7. Explain the changes observed in the EEG as the severity of an ischemic attack in the brain progresses.

8. What are the basic features of the EEG?

9. What is the typical amplitude range of the EEG?

10. What range of EEG frequencies are clinically useful?

11. Give the names and the frequency range of the four typical EEG bands.

12. What is the distribution of EEG frequencies on the head of an awake normal adult?

13. What is the typical EEG pattern observed in a normal adult under anesthesia?

14. What is the minimum montage adequate for intraoperative EEG monitoring?

15. What are the recommended cutoff settings for the high frequency and low frequency filters during intraoperative EEG monitoring?

16. What kind of changes does a localized ischemic cortical attack have on the EEG?

17. How do EEG changes due to an ischemic attack differ from EEG changes due to modifications in anesthesia regime?

18. What is an EMG?

19. Can the frequency of stimulation of a muscle change the strength of muscle contraction? Explain.

20. What is the clinical use of the EMG?

21. What is the main advantage of EMG compared to SEP monitoring in spine surgery?

22. What is the main objective of EMG monitoring?

23. What is the primary criterion used for intraoperative interpretation of EMG recording?

24. Is it possible to monitor all 12 cranial nerves using EMG? Explain.

25. Name the muscles used to monitor the fifth and seventh cranial nerves.

26. Which cranial nerves can monitor from the trapezius muscle and the tongue?

27. When stimulating only one spinal root in the lumbar area, is it possible to detect responses in more than one muscle? Explain.

28. Name the muscles used for monitoring the spinal roots from L_2 to S_3 levels.

29. What is the most important factor affecting EMG monitoring?

30. How is level of relaxation typically determined?

31. What does it mean for a patient to be "reversed"?

32. What are the interpretation criteria for possible nerve injury?

chapter 7

Evoked Activity

7.1 Introduction

A clinically important tool in assessing the integrity of cortical and subcortical neuronal relays is the study of evoked responses (ERs) which result from external stimulation of a neural pathway.

The rationale for using ERs intraoperatively is very simple: all naturally occurring
external stimuli detected by the sense organs, such as sounds and lights, are transmitted
to the brain in the form of electrical signals through various sensory neural pathways.
If these pathways are structurally and functionally intact, the signals reaching the brain
give rise to certain patterns of activity. Thus, like the natural stimuli, the delivery
of experimental stimuli, such as tones or electrical pulses, and the simultaneous
observation of the resulting patterns of activity provide an instantaneous display of
the status of the sensory neural structures intervening between the stimulation and
recording sites.

ERs can be subdivided further into *averaged* and *nonaveraged* responses, examples
of which are the familiar evoked potentials (EPs) and the electrically triggered EMG,
respectively. In this chapter we present details on the use, features, stimulation, and
recording procedures, as well as interpretation criteria of the various kinds of averaged
and nonaveraged ERs.

7.2 Evoked Potentials

An EP is the electrical response of the nervous system to external stimulation. There
are two major types of EPs, *sensory* and *motor*. In the former category, a stimulus
is delivered peripherally (e.g., at a leg nerve) and the resulting response is recorded
centrally (e.g., the cortex). In the latter category, a stimulus is delivered centrally
(e.g., at the cortex) and the resulting response is recorded peripherally (e.g., at a leg
nerve or muscle).

Depending on the stimulus modality, sensory EPs are divided into *somatosensory,*
auditory, and *visual,* indicated as SEPs, AEPs, and VEPs, respectively. Early AEPs
are referred to as *brainstem auditory evoked responses* (BAERs). Motor EPs can be

further divided into *neurogenic* and *myogenic,* depending on whether the response is recorded at a nerve or at a muscle.

Single-trial evoked responses are not readily apparent in the background activity and, to detect them, averaging of several trials is necessary (see Section 4.4.10). The averaged EPs consist of an ordered series of negative or positive components (waves or peaks) of particular morphology, amplitude, and latency. These three characteristics are the variables to be monitored intraoperatively.

For averaged responses, regardless of the stimulus modality, the *stimulation rate* should be relatively high, so that data are collected fast enough and average responses are updated sufficiently often to allow early detection of possible response changes. However, this rate should not exceed a certain critical value, to avoid degradation of response amplitude and morphology. Moreover, the interval between successive stimuli should not match the period of any oscillatory signals, such as the well-known 60 Hz power-line cycle, otherwise the averaged responses will contain a periodic artifact. To avoid this synchronization problem, a noninteger stimulation rate should be used, such as, for instance, 4.7 Hz.

Also, in all modalities the *analysis time* or *time base,* that is, the length (in msec) of the segment of signal collected following each stimulus, is another factor to consider in selecting the stimulation rate. If the interval between successive stimuli is shorter than the analysis time, a stimulus artifact will be present in the averaged response. The analysis time is selected so that all peaks of interest fall within the analysis window.

During the course of surgery, ongoing responses (the last set of EPs) are compared against a set of *baselines* which are obtained *after* induction of anesthesia and final positioning of the patient and *before* any surgical manipulation. However, if after the incision and before any surgical maneuvering, the responses have changed excessively due, for example, to drastic changes in anesthesia regime, such as use of different anesthetic agents or induction of hypotension, then the baselines should be reestablished.

Baseline recordings should be of familiar morphology, should contain clear and reliable components, and should also be consistent with the clinical picture of the patient. However, one should keep in mind that the purpose of intraoperative monitoring is to detect response *changes due to surgery, not to make a clinical diagnosis.* Baselines should remain on the screen for comparison with the current responses throughout the case.

Like the ongoing activity presented in Chapter 6, evoked responses are affected by anesthetic agents, blood pressure, and body temperature, since all these factors can alter blood perfusion and metabolic rate in neural cells. In the following sections we concentrate on different types of evoked activity typically recorded during the course of neurological, orthopedic, or vascular surgery and we give details regarding the generation, information content, recommended electrode locations, and typical acquisition parameters. A quick summary of the various factors that affect the recorded neurophysiological signals, such as pharmacological agents and induced neuroprotective conditions, is also presented, along with information to assist with the interpretation of the results.

7.3   Somatosensory Evoked Potentials

7.3.1   Generation

Somatosensory evoked potentials (SEPs) can be elicited by electrical stimulation of
a peripheral nerve, such as the median nerve at the wrist or the posterior tibial nerve
at the ankle. The location of these nerves is schematically shown in Figure 7.1.

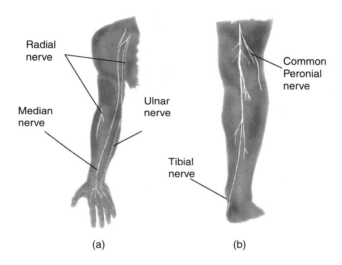

Figure 7.1   Schematic diagram of (a) the median nerve at the wrist and (b) the posterior tibial
nerve at the ankle.

These nerves are part of the somatosensory system, a schematic diagram of which
is shown in Figure 7.2. Evoked activity travels along the stimulated nerve and enters
the spinal cord through the dorsal roots. From there, ascending pathways take the
impulses first to the brainstem, then to the thalamus and, finally, to the primary sensory
cortex. Ascending volleys of SEPs can be recorded at any point along this pathway.

More specifically, activity within the spinal cord is conveyed by the dorsomedial
tracts, and remains ipsilateral to its side of entry. A first synapse is formed in the
medulla, the inferior portion of the brainstem, in the *nucleus gracilis* for fibers from the
lower portion of the body and in the *nucleus cuneatus* for fibers from the upper portion
of the body. Fibers leaving the medulla decussate to form the contralateral *medial
lemniscus* and terminate in the thalamus, where a second synapse is formed. Fibers
leaving the thalamus terminate in the sensory cortex in a somatotopic arrangement.
Legs are represented close to the midline, whereas arms and hands are represented
more laterally. A diagram of the somatotopic arrangement of the primary sensory
cortex is shown in Figure 7.3.

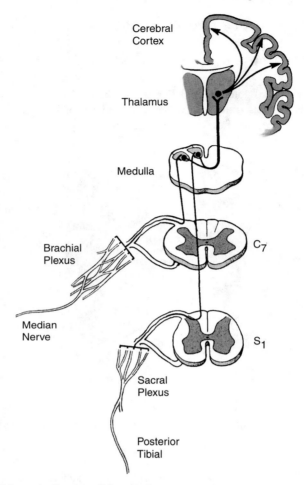

Figure 7.2   Schematic diagram of the somatosensory system.

7.3.2   *Use*

Somatosensory evoked potentials are used intraoperatively to:

- Monitor blood perfusion of the cortex or the spinal cord (e.g., during an aneurysm clipping).

- Monitor the structural and functional integrity of the spinal cord during ortho-pedic or neurological surgery (e.g., for scoliosis or a spinal tumor).

- Monitor structural and functional integrity of peripheral nerves (e.g., sciatic nerve during ascetabular fixation), spinal nerve roots (e.g., during decom-pression in radiculopathy), and peripheral nerve structures (e.g., the brachial plexus).

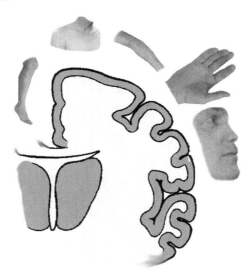

Figure 7.3   Somatotopic arrangement of the primary sensory cortex showing the "homunculus."

- Determine *functional* identity of cortical tissue (e.g., one can separate the sensory from motor cortex by identifying the central sulcus).

7.3.3   SEP Features

In general, monitoring protocols require stimulation of the left and right sides of the body independently, resulting in two sets of responses, one from each side. Typical recordings include a peripheral, a subcortical, and a cortical response. The peripheral response is typically recorded from the Erb's point for arm stimulation, or the popliteal fossa for leg stimulation. The two central responses are obtained from a cervical and a cortical location, respectively. The locations of the stimulating and recording electrodes are schematically shown in Figures 7.4 and 7.5 for arm and leg stimulation, respectively.

Normal SEPs consist of clear, reliable, and bilaterally symmetric components. That is, the waveforms obtained have standard, known morphology, and the individual peaks are clearly identifiable against the background (noise-free recordings). Additionally, repeated recordings from the same limb result in similar (within 10%) amplitudes and latencies. Similarly, the difference in amplitude and latency between the two limbs is minimal (typically, less than 10%).

7.3.4   Recording Procedure

The choice for the peripheral nerve to stimulate depends on the site of surgery [54]. Typically, if the site of surgery is (1) above the level of the seventh cervical vertebra (Cvii), one should stimulate the median nerve; (2) above and including the level of

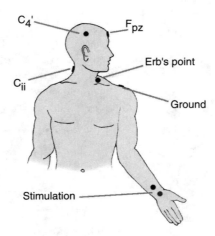

Figure 7.4   Location of the stimulating and recording electrodes to record median nerve SEPs.

Cvii, the ulnar nerve; and (3) below Cvii, the posterior tibial nerve. It is recommended, however, to always monitor brachial plexus function, through ulnar nerve stimulation, to avoid a possible plexopathy from improper positioning of a patient's shoulders.

Stimulation Parameters

Electrical stimulation of a peripheral nerve is commonly used to elicit somatosensory responses which can be recorded from the spinal cord or the brain. The number of fibers excited by an electrical stimulus is determined by the amount of current delivered. *Constant current* stimulation results in more stable responses, because the number of fibers excited with each stimulus remains the same.

The *intensity* and *duration* of the stimuli are adjusted so that the stimulation achieved is supramaximal [54, 66], that is, all neuronal axons are forced to fire. However, care should be taken to avoid skin damage and local burns from stimuli of excessively high intensity or long duration. Typical intensity values are 25 mA for arm stimulation and 50 mA for leg stimulation. The stimulus duration is set at 0.3 msec in both cases [57].

As explained in Section 7.2, a noninteger stimulation rate, such as 4.7 Hz, is used to avoid synchronization with power line interference. A time base of 100 msec is sufficient to produce reliable responses with all peaks falling within the analysis window [20].

Recording Parameters

When recording cortical responses, which represent mostly activity on neuronal dendrites, a bandwidth between 10 and 300 Hz is required, whereas for subcortical activity, which is primarily due to axonal sources, a frequency range between 10

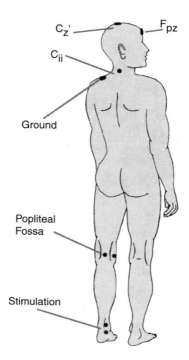

Figure 7.5   Location of the stimulating and recording electrodes to record posterior tibial nerve SEPs.

and 3000 Hz is necessary. Reliable SEPs can be obtained with 300 trials for arm stimulation and 500 trials for leg stimulation [54].

Recording Sites

The somatotopic arrangement of the sensory cortex should be kept in mind when recording SEPs. The electrodes are placed on the scalp on specific locations in order to obtain maximum responses to sensory stimuli, according to the 10–20 international placement system used in clinical applications. The typical electrode locations for recording median nerve SEPs are shown in Figure 7.6(a), where arrows indicate the recording montage. For simplicity, only the channels corresponding to right-hand stimulation are shown.

Similarly, typical electrode locations for recording posterior tibial nerve SEPs are shown in Figure 7.6(b). In this case, an additional channel, not shown in Figure 7.6(b), is used for the recording from the popliteal fossa. Electrode C_3', C_4', and C_z' are placed 2 cm behind C_3, C_4, and C_z, respectively. Table 7.1 summarizes the acquisition parameters recommended for intraoperative monitoring of median and posterior tibial nerve SEPs, respectively.

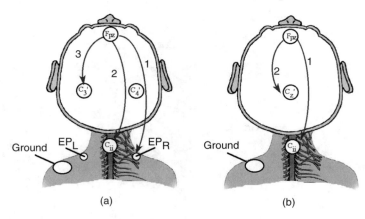

Figure 7.6 Typical electrode locations for intraoperative recordings of (a) median nerve and (b) posterior tibial nerve SEPs.

Table 7.1 Recommended Parameter Settings for Recording Median and Posterior Tibial Nerve SEPs

Side	Recording		Stimulation			Time Base	Sensitivity
(stim)	Channel	Bandwidth	Intensity	Rate	Duration		
			Median Nerve				
Left	$F_{pz}-C_4'$	10–300 Hz					
	$F_{pz}-C_{ii}$						
	$F_{pz}-EP_L$	20–2000 Hz	25 mA	4.7 Hz	0.3 msec	100 msec	10 μV
Right	$F_{pz}-C_3'$	10–300 Hz					
	$F_{pz}-C_{ii}$						
	$F_{pz}-EP_R$	10–2000 Hz					
			Posterior Tibial Nerve				
Left	$F_{pz}-C_z'$	10–300 Hz					
	$F_{pz}-C_{ii}$						
	PF_L	10–2000 Hz	50 mA	4.7 Hz	0.3 msec	100 msec	10 μV
Right	$F_{pz}-C_z'$	10–300 Hz					
	$F_{pz}-C_{ii}$						
	PF_R	10–2000 Hz					

7.3.5   SEPs to Arm Stimulation

A common technique is to stimulate the median nerve at the wrist[1] while recording along the nerve pathway, initially from Erb's point, a clavicular location shown in Figure 7.7, then from a cervical point at the level of the second vertebra (C_{ii}), and finally from the contralateral parietal cortex (C_3' or C_4').

---

[1]As explained in Section 3.5.2, the negative stimulating electrode is always placed closer to the recording side.

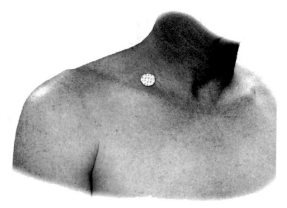

Figure 7.7   Anatomic location of Erb's point.

When the wrist is not accessible, as when, for example, the patient's arm is in a cast, the median nerve can be stimulated at alternate sites, namely at the elbow or the axilla. The correct locations for placing the stimulating electrodes at the wrist, elbow, and axilla are shown in Figure 7.8.

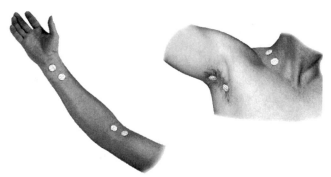

Figure 7.8   Placement of stimulating electrodes along the median nerve pathway.

Similar responses are detected from ulnar or radial nerve stimulation, although the amplitude of individual peaks is lower, apparently due to a smaller number of fibers being activated [66]. Figure 7.9 shows the correct sites for placing the stimulation electrodes along the pathway of the ulnar nerve at the wrist and at the elbow.

To record SEPs, the active (negative) electrodes are placed over the Erb's point, the cervical C_{ii} vertebra, and the C_3' and C_4' locations on the scalp. Electrode C_3' and C_4' are placed 2 cm behind C_3 and C_4, respectively. The inactive (positive) electrode is placed on the forehead (F_{pz}) [20] with a ground on a shoulder.

Approximately 9 msec after stimulation of the median nerve at the wrist the Erb's point electrode detects a negative component (N9), which represents action potentials generated by the peripheral nerve fibers contained in the brachial plexus [9]. About

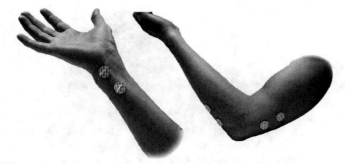

Figure 7.9   Placement of stimulating electrodes along the ulnar nerve pathway.

13 msec following stimulation the cervical electrode detects a major negative component (N13), which is generated probably by several sources in the dorsal column of the spinal cord. This component is presumably made up of both excitatory postsynaptic potentials and action potentials. The most important scalp-recorded component has a negative peak at about 20 msec which is followed by a positive peak at about 25 msec, forming the N20–P25 complex. The N20 probably originates from the parietal sensory cortical area contralateral to the side of stimulation [66].

An example of typical components obtained along the sensory pathway after stimulation of the median nerve at the wrist is shown in Figure 7.10. Notice the symmetry of the responses obtained on the left and right sides.

7.3.6   SEPs to Leg Stimulation

SEPs to leg stimulation can be obtained by stimulating the posterior tibial nerve at the ankle while recording peripherally from the popliteal fossa, and from cervical and scalp electrodes.

When the ankle is not accessible, as when, for example, the patient's leg is in a cast, the posterior tibial nerve can be stimulated at the popliteal fossa. The correct placement of the stimulating electrodes along the pathway of the posterior tibial nerve is shown in Figure 7.11.

Similar responses are detected from peroneal nerve stimulation, although the amplitude of individual peaks is lower. Figure 7.12 shows the correct sites for placing the stimulation electrodes along the pathway of the peroneal nerve.

To record SEPs, the active (negative) electrode for the peripheral response is placed above the popliteal crease, whereas the inactive (positive) electrode is placed on the medial surface of the knee. The cervical and cortical responses can be obtained by placing the active (negative) electrode over C_{ii} and C_z', respectively, whereas the inactive (positive) electrode for both responses is placed on the forehead (F_{pz}).

The popliteal fossa response consists of a negative component (N9) with latency approximately 9 msec, and it is generated by the peripheral nerve fibers [9, 66]. The cervical component (N30) has a latency of approximately 30 msec and probably reflects activity of nuclei in the dorsal column of the spinal cord. The most prominent cortical component has a positive peak at about 37 msec and is followed by a negative

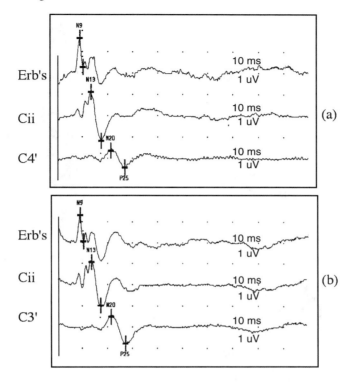

Figure 7.10   Typical components obtained after stimulation of the median nerve at the (a) left and (b) right wrist.

peak at about 45 msec, forming the P37–N45 complex. The actual normal latency values vary considerably with patient height and other factors [66].

An example of typical components obtained along the sensory pathway after stimulation of the posterior tibial nerve at the ankle is shown in Figure 7.13. Similar peaks are detected from common peroneal nerve stimulation at the knee but, since the total length of the neural pathway is shorter, the latencies of the cervical and cortical components are shorter by about 10 msec.

7.3.7   *Affecting Factors*

Inhaled Anesthetic Agents

Nitrous oxide (N_2O) reduces the amplitude and increases the latency of cortical components in a dose-dependent fashion [43].

Inhalational anesthetics, such as *Isoflurane, Halothane,* and *Enflurane,* all decrease the amplitude and increase the latency of the cortical responses in a dose-dependent fashion, especially when they are administered with N_2O [43].

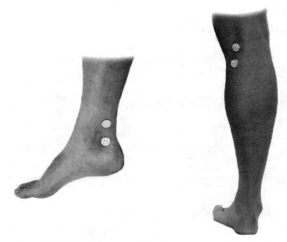

Figure 7.11   Placement of stimulating electrodes along the posterior tibial nerve pathway.

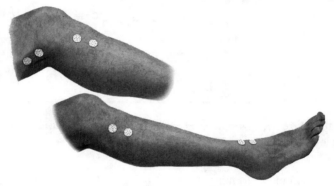

Figure 7.12   Placement of stimulating electrodes along the peroneal nerve pathway.

Intravenous Agents

Propofol does not affect the subcortical N13 component, but it increases the latency by approximately 10% of the early cortical components without affecting their amplitude. Later cortical components usually disappear [43].

Benzodiazepines (e.g., Diazepam, Midazolam) reduce the amplitude of cortical SEP waves [42].

Barbiturates (e.g., Thiopental, Methohexital) increase SEP latency in a dose-dependent fashion, with a slight amplitude decrease [43].

Etomidate has a surprising effect on the cortical SEP amplitude, which can be augmented by as much as 200–600% [43]. However, it also increases SEP latencies.

Ketamine also increases SEP amplitude and latency [43, 21].

Opiates, such as Morphine, and synthetic narcotics, such as Fentanyl, Alfentanil, and Sufentanil, cause a slight increase in SEP latency without affecting the amplitude [42].

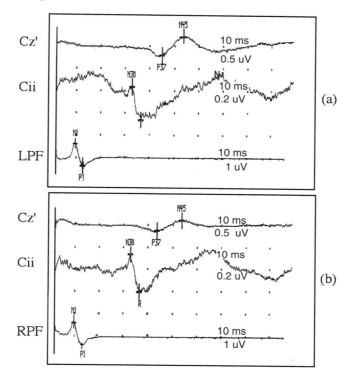

Figure 7.13 Typical components obtained after stimulation of the posterior tibial nerve at the (a) left and (b) right ankle.

Muscle relaxants, such as Saccinycholine, Pancuronium, and Vecuronium, do not affect SEPs directly. However, they may improve SEP amplitude by reducing background muscle activity.

In general, narcotics can be administered either as bolus injection or drip infusion. The former method will typically result in a drastic reduction of the cortical SEP amplitude for about 15 min following the injection. On the other hand, drip infusion of the same agent has minimal effects on SEPs. Therefore, for proper intraoperative monitoring the latter method is preferred. Table 7.2 summarizes the effects of various drugs most commonly used in anesthesia on the cortical SEPs.

Induced Conditions

Hypotension, induced by Nitroprusside in typical doses, has a minimal direct effect on SEPs. However, severe hypotension (mean arterial pressure 50 mmHg or less) results in a drastic decrease or even total loss of the cervical and cortical responses.

Hypothermia increases the latency and may slightly decrease the amplitude of SEPs. *Hyperthermia* will decrease the latency of the responses by about 5% per 1°C, and may also decrease their amplitude slightly.

Table 7.2   Effects of Anesthetic Agents on Cortical SEP Amplitude
and Latency

Agent	Amplitude	Latency
Nitrous Oxide (N₂O)	⇓	⇒
Inhalational Anesthetics Isoflurane, Halothane, Enflurane, Desflurane	⇓	⇒
Propofol	—	→
Barbiturates Thiopental, Methohexital	↓	⇒
Etomidate	⇓	→
Ketamine	⇓	→
Opiates Morphine, Fentanyl, Alfentanil, Sufentanil	—	→
Benzodiazepines Diazepam, Midazolam	⇓	⇒
Muscle Relaxants Saccinycholine, Pancuronium, Vecuronium	—	—
Hypotensive Agents Nitroprusside, Nitroglycerine	↓	→

Note: Modest (↓) or significant (⇑ or ⇓) amplitude change; —: no change.
Modest (→) or significant (⇒) latency increase.

Age

Newborn babies often show a cortical N30 component after stimulation of arm nerves
and a P50 after stimulation of leg nerves [66]. SEPs gradually reach adult form and
latencies at an age between 3 and 10 years. In older adults (>60 years), the amplitude
of SEPs decreases slightly, whereas the latency increases progressively with age,
especially in the cortical components, due to decreased peripheral conduction velocity
with age [66].

Limb Length

Since absolute latencies depend on the distance between the stimulating and the
recording electrodes, it is expected that longer limbs will introduce a slight latency
increase [66].

7.3.8   SEP Intraoperative Interpretation

Typical amplitude and latency values for normal SEP components are reported in Table 7.3.

Table 7.3   Typical SEP Amplitude and Latency Values
Obtained After Median or Posterior Tibial Nerve Stimulation

Nerve	Site	Peak	Amplitude μV	Latency msec
	Erb's Point	N9	1.6	9
Median	Cervical	N13	1.5	13
	Cortical	N20	0.9	21
		P25		27
Posterior	Popliteal Fossa	N9	1.5	10
Tibial	Cervical	N30	0.3	32
	Cortical	P37	0.7	43
		N45		52

After induction and final positioning of the patient, a set of baselines is obtained which remains on the screen for comparison throughout the case. Baseline responses should be of familiar morphology and contain clear and reliable components. The baselines should also be consistent with the clinical picture of the patient.

During surgery, interpretation criteria are based on detection of reliable and significant changes compared to the baselines established at the beginning of the case. Changes mainly involve the amplitude and latency of the SEP components recorded at different levels. A change is *reliable* if it is repeatable at least twice in a row; and it is *significant* if the amplitude has decreased by at least 50% or the latency has increased by at least 10% [35, 54].

As explained earlier, changes in amplitude and/or latency can result also from perisurgical factors. Hence, successful differentiation of SEP changes due to iatrogenic factors is based on (1) evaluation of the change pattern (e.g., a sudden change vs. a gradual change, or a change that affected the cortical component only vs. a change that affected also the peripheral response); and (2) correlation of the change pattern with surgical maneuvers, blood pressure, oxygen saturation, administration of drugs, and body temperature.

In general, SEP changes due to surgical maneuvers (e.g., spinal distraction) or ischemia (e.g., after placement of an artery clamp) are abrupt and localized (i.e., only one side of the body may be affected), whereas changes due to anesthesia or body temperature changes and bolus injection of drugs are relatively slower and generalized.

Table 7.4 summarizes the SEP changes that can be observed at various recording levels, a plausible interpretation, and the recommended action to take.

Table 7.4 Summary of Possible SEP Changes During Intraoperative Monitoring, Interpretation, and Possible Actions

Peripheral	Cervical	Cortical	Interpretation	Action
OK	OK	OK	Normal	None
		⇊	Anesthesia change	Contact anesthesiologist
OK	OK	⇒ Ø	Anesthesia change or cortical ischemia	Contact anesthesiologist Contact surgeon
OK	⇊ Ø	OK	Muscle activity artifact or faulty recording electrode or amplifier turned off	Contact anesthesiologist Check/change electrode Check amplifier
OK	⇊ ⇒ Ø	⇊ ⇒ Ø	Mechanical insult or spinal cord ischemia	Contact surgeon Contact anesthesiologist
⇊ Ø	OK	OK	Faulty recording electrode or amplifier turned off	Check/change electrode Check amplifier
⇊	OK	⇊ ⇒ Ø		Check/change electrode Check amplifier
⇊	⇊	OK	Muscle activity artifact	Contact anesthesiologist
⇊ ⇒	⇊ ⇒	⇊ ⇒	Systemic change or peripheral nerve ischemia	Contact surgeon Contact anesthesiologist
⇊ Ø	⇊ Ø	⇊ Ø	Faulty stimulating electrode or faulty stimulating device	Check/change electrode Check stimulating device

Note: OK: no change; ⇊: amplitude decrease; ⇒ latency increase; Ø: no response present.

7.4   DSEPs

7.4.1   Generation

Dermatomes are areas of skin supplied by cutaneous branches of spinal nerves. Dermatomal somatosensory evoked potentials (DSEPs) are elicited by stimulation of specific dermatomal fields. Elicited activity travels along the same pathways described in the SEP section. Since the exact cutaneous distribution of dermatomes is still debated, the stimulation sites used are those most commonly accepted. Figure 7.14 shows a diagram with the distribution of dermatomes over the arm and leg.

7.4.2   Use

DSEPs are used intraoperatively during procedures in which nerve root rather than spinal cord function is at risk, for example, during lumbar spine surgery for root decompression. Since the input of peripheral nerves into the spinal cord is spread over several levels (spinal roots), SEPs do not provide information about the integrity of single nerve roots. Thus, an abnormality at one level may result in a small (within normal limits) variation of activity and be obscured by an overall apparent upkeep of normal activity. On the contrary, DSEPs provide information that is root-specific [55, 71].

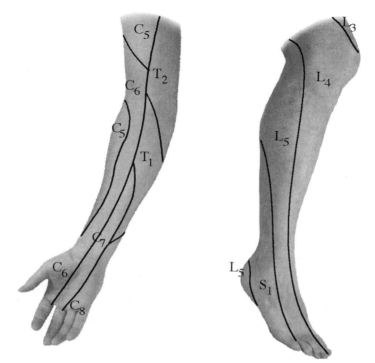

Figure 7.14   Distribution of dermatomes over the arm and the leg.

7.4.3   DSEP Features

DSEPs have the same amplitude and latency features as SEPs. However, dermatomal stimulation yields components of smaller amplitude and increased latency, since the excited nerve fibers are smaller and fewer in number [18, 54, 71]. For the same reason DSEPs are more difficult to record than SEPs, especially from noncephalic electrodes.

7.4.4   Recording Procedure

Stimulation Parameters

The electrodes for cutaneous stimulation are placed a few centimeters apart within the same dermatome. The stimulus intensity is submaximal, i.e., about 2 to 3 times that of the sensory threshold, to avoid stimulation of the underlying tissue [18, 55]. A stimulation rate of 4.7 Hz, with a stimulus duration of 0.3 msec, is used. The low and high filters are set at 10 and 300 Hz, respectively. Clear and reliable responses can be obtained with approximately 500 single trials. Each side should be stimulated independently. The most common stimulation sites are dermatomes L_3, L_4, L_5, and S_1.

Recording Sites

When recording DSEPs, the somatotopic arrangement of the sensory cortex should be kept in mind. The active (negative) electrodes are placed over the somatosensory cortex at the standard C'_3, C'_4, and C'_z locations, whereas the inactive (positive) electrode is placed on the forehead (F_{pz}). The ground electrode is placed on the patient's shoulder. The peripheral and cervical responses are usually unclear and typically not recorded.

7.4.5   Affecting Factors

DSEPs are affected by the same factors affecting SEPs.

7.4.6   DSEP Intraoperative Interpretation

Soon after induction and final positioning of the patient, a set of baselines is obtained which remains on the screen for comparison throughout the case. Baseline responses should be of familiar morphology and contain clear and reliable components. The baselines should also be consistent with the clinical picture of the patient.

Normal DSEPs from the same limb should show about 3 msec of latency difference from one level to the next. Additionally, the maximum latency difference between the two limbs should be less than about 6 msec [54].

Interpretation of DSEPs follows the same guidelines as SEPs. However, the most significant DSEP feature is latency, not amplitude. Small latency shifts, as low as 4%, may be significant and may indicate a potential root injury [18].

Also, since DSEPs show abnormalities before surgery, responses usually improve during surgery. However, although the amount of improvement and adequacy of decompression are correlated, the former does not necessarily constitute an absolute indicator of the latter.

7.5   Brainstem Auditory Evoked Responses

7.5.1   Generation

Brainstem auditory evoked responses (BAERs) are elicited by auditory stimulation and represent activity generated in the VIII cranial nerve and brainstem structures in the rostral medulla, pons and caudal midbrain [46]. Typically, BAERs consist of five clear waves or peaks (indicated as peak I, II, III, IV, and V), all occurring within the first 10 msec after stimulus onset. Often, peak VI and VII are also well defined. Each peak presumably has a specific origin along the auditory pathway, mainly ipsilateral to the stimulated ear. Figure 7.15 shows the first five peaks seen in a typical BAER waveform.

The putative sites of origin for wave I and II are the extracranial and intracranial portions of the cochlear nerve, respectively [46]. Wave III is most likely generated in the ipsilateral cochlear nucleus, whereas wave IV and V are generated in multiple brainstem sites and do not bear a one-to-one relationship to any particular struc-

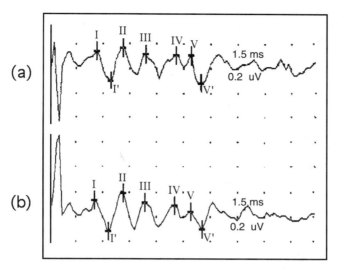

Figure 7.15   Typical BAER waveform obtained after ipsilateral stimulation of the (a) left and (b) right ear, showing peaks I through V.

tures [48]. Most likely, peaks VI and VII are of cortical origin. Figure 7.16 depicts the commonly accepted generators along the primary auditory pathway.

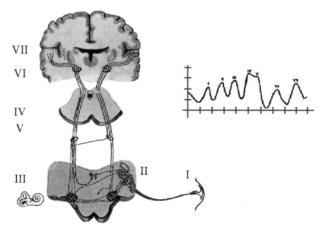

Figure 7.16   Putative sites of origin of the first few BAER wave.

7.5.2   Use

BAERs are used intraoperatively to assess the functional integrity of acoustic pathway structures, particularly those located in the brainstem. Typical situations requiring

BAER monitoring include surgery for acoustic tumors, and procedures involving the cerebello-pontine angle and the posterior fossa.

7.5.3   BAER Features

The basic BAER features used for intraoperative analysis include measurement of peak amplitudes, as well as peak and interpeak latencies [46, 20]. Occasionally, normal recordings may not contain all of the peaks. Wave V is the most reliable one and is present most of the times, along with wave I and III. Wave II is often missing, whereas wave IV may partially or completely merge with wave V [66].

If peak I is unclear, its amplitude may be increased by increasing the stimulus intensity and possibly decreasing the stimulation rate. The main difference between ipsilateral and contralateral BAER is in peak I, which is unclear or absent in the contralateral recording [66]. Typical amplitude and latency values for peaks I through V are reported in Table 7.5.

Table 7.5   Typical BAER Amplitude and Latency Values and Interpeak Latency Differences for Peaks I Through V

Wave	Amplitude	Latency	Interpeak Latency	
I	0.2	1.7	I–III	2.1
II		2.8	III–V	1.9
III		3.9	I–V	4.0
IV		5.1		
V	0.5	5.7		

7.5.4   Recording Procedure

Recording Sites

Proper intraoperative monitoring for evaluation of acoustic nerve and brainstem function requires that each ear be stimulated independently. Therefore, it is necessary to use two recording channels, one for each ear. The active (negative) electrode is placed on the earlobe ipsilateral to the side of stimulation (A_1 or A_2), whereas the reference (positive) electrode is placed on the vertex (C_z). The ground electrode is located on the forehead (F_{pz}) [66, 75]. An example of such an arrangement is shown in Figure 7.17.

This montage allows to compare activity on the affected site with activity on the homotopic unaffected site as it propagates along the auditory pathway. However, it is possible to make use of bilateral stimulation, when both ears are stimulated simultaneously, if the peaks to unilateral stimulation are not clear or reliable.

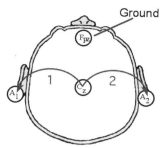

Figure 7.17   BAER recording protocol.

Stimulation Approach

Auditory stimulation, commonly consists of series of clicks, which are usually delivered through foam ear inserts attached to air tube. The latter are connected to sound generators located away from the patient's head. The tubes introduce a latency delay in all peaks (typical value 1 msec) which, depending on the recording system, may or may not be accounted for automatically by the software. Reliable BAERs are obtained after delivery of *rarefaction* rather than *condensation* click stimuli, in which case the tympanic membrane moves away from the ear. These stimuli produce sudden excitation and result in well-defined peaks [44, 46, 75].

A stimulus intensity of approximately 80 dB nHL[2] delivered at a noninteger rate, e.g., 11.1 Hz, is sufficient to elicit reliable BAERs and avoid synchronization with interfering electrical noise. Each stimulus should have a duration between 0.03 and 0.1 msec. When the stimulus is applied to one ear, the sound is conducted through the skull and may reach the opposite ear. This effect can be avoided by applying a constant masking stimulus (typically white noise) to the contralateral ear. The noise intensity should be about 40 dB below the stimulus intensity [20, 66].

Approximately 1200 to 1500 single trials are sufficient for reliable averaged responses, although in certain cases this number must be increased. An analysis time of 10 msec allows for all peaks of interest to fall within the observation window. Filter settings should allow all frequencies between 30 and 3000 Hz to be recorded [46, 66]. Table 7.6 summarizes the recommended acquisition parameters for BAERs.

Table 7.6   Recommended Parameter Settings for Recording BAERs

Ear	Recording			Stimulus			Time
	Channel	Bandwidth	Sensitivity	Type	Intensity	Polarity	Base
Left	$C_z–A_1$			Click	80 dB		
	$C_z–A_2$	30–3000 Hz	1 μV	Noise	40 dB	Rarefaction	10 msec
Right	$C_z–A_1$			Noise	40 dB		
	$C_z–A_2$			Click	80 dB		

[2]*Normal hearing level* (nHL) is the average threshold intensity of normal hearing young adults for a specific type of stimuli, such as clicks, and it is measured in decibels (dB).

7.5.5   Affecting Factors

Inhalational Anesthetic Agents

Nitrous oxide (N$_2$O) results in a linear decrease of BAER amplitude with no change in latency [42].

Isoflurane, Halothane, and *Enflurane* mildly increase BAER latencies [42].

Intravenous Agents

Propofol increases the latency of peaks I, II, and V, but it does not affect their amplitude [42].

Barbiturates (e.g., Thiopental, Methohexital) and *Ketamine* increase BAER interpeak latency [21].

Fentanyl and other narcotics even in large doses have minimal effect in BAERs [42].

Benzodiazepines (e.g., Diazepam, Midazolam) have minimal effect in BAERs [21].

Induced Conditions

Hypothermia increases the latency and decreases the amplitude BAERs [21, 66], whereas *hyperthermia* decreases the amplitude [42] and the latency [21] of the responses. In general, BAER latencies are inversely related to temperature at a rate of about 0.2 msec/°C.

Muscle relaxants, such as Saccinycholine, Pancuronium and Vecuronium, have no effect on BAERs.

In general, most anesthetic agents in typical doses will have only minimal effects on BAERs [20], as shown in Table 7.7.

7.5.6   BAER Intraoperative Interpretation

Typically, after induction and final positioning of the patient, a set of baselines is obtained which remains on the screen for comparison throughout the case. Baseline responses should contain clear and reliable components, and should also be correlated with the clinical picture of the patient. For example, peripheral hearing loss may result in unclear or absent peaks.

During surgery, BAER interpretation criteria are based on the detection of significant changes, compared to the baselines, mainly in the amplitude and latency of peaks I and V, as well as the interpeak latencies from peak I to III and from III to V. These interpeak latencies represent the peripheral and central conduction time, respectively. BAERs are subcortical in origin and, thus, little affected by anesthetics or small changes in the anesthesia regime [20]. Therefore, even small changes may be significant. Traditionally, the most important criterion involves the latency and the amplitude of peak V [48]. A change repeated twice in a row must be reported even if the latency has increased by only 0.5 msec. A shift of 1–1.5 msec usually indicates that some action must be taken [48].

Table 7.7   Effects of Anesthetic Agents on BAER Amplitude and Latency

Agent	Amplitude	Latency
Nitrous Oxide (N_2O)	↓	—
Inhalational Anesthetics Isoflurane, Halothane, Enflurane, Desflurane	—	→
Propofol	—	→
Barbiturates Thiopental, Methohexital	—	→
Ketamine	—	→
Opiates Morphine, Fentanyl, Alfentanil, Sufentanil	—	—
Benzodiazepines Diazepam, Midazolam	—	—
Muscle Relaxants Saccinycholine, Pancuronium, Vecuronium	—	—

Note: Modest (↓) amplitude change; —: no change. Modest (→) latency increase.

7.6   Visual Evoked Potentials

7.6.1   Generation

Visual evoked potentials (VEPs) result from stimulation of the visual pathway. Activity generated in the retina leaves the eye through the *optic nerve.* The two optic nerves, one from each eye, join at the *optic chiasm* where fibers from the nasal half of each retina cross to the opposite side, while fibers from the temporal half do not cross. This fiber segregation results into two *optic tracts,* each containing a complete representation of the contralateral hemifield of vision. The optic tracts terminate in the thalamus and other subcortical structures. From there, through the *optic radiations,* activity reaches the primary visual cortex in the occipital lobes. The gross anatomy of the visual system is depicted in Figure 7.18.

7.6.2   Use

VEPs are used intraoperatively to assess the functional integrity of the visual pathway during surgery for tumors or trauma involving the optic nerves, chiasm, optic tracts, and the occipital visual cortex. VEPs are most useful in cases involving the retro-orbital and parasellar regions [20, 48, 69] (see also Figure 9.4).

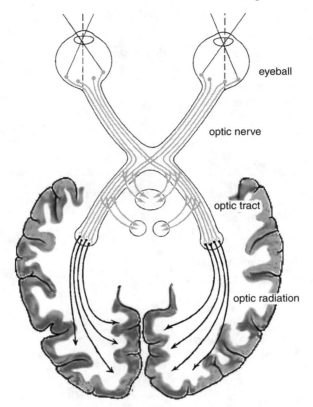

Figure 7.18   Gross anatomy of the visual system.

7.6.3   VEP Features

Intraoperative analysis of VEP features involves measurement of peak amplitudes, as well as peak and interpeak latencies. Typical flash VEPs contain two major positive components, P_1 and P_2, found at about 100 and 170 msec after stimulus onset, respectively. Each of the components is preceded by a negative one, N_1 and N_2, at about 70 and 140 msec, respectively. The latter components however are less clear and stable. All components are generated by the visual cortex [20]. Figure 7.19 shows a typical VEP waveform.

7.6.4   Recording Procedure

Recording Sites

A typical montage for intraoperative monitoring includes two recording channels, each involving one hemisphere. The active (positive) electrodes are placed on the O_1 an O_2 standard EEG locations, whereas the inactive (negative) electrodes are placed on the contralateral earlobe (A_2 and A_1, respectively). Alternatively, a vertex (C_z)

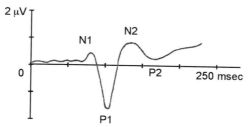

Figure 7.19   Typical VEPs obtained from flash stimulation.

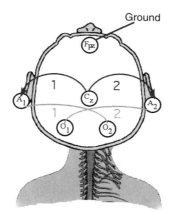

Figure 7.20   Two alternative montages for recording VEPs.

electrode can be used as a reference for both channels. The ground is placed on the forehead (F_{pz}). An example of such an arrangement is shown in Figure 7.20.

Stimulation Approach

Flash stimuli are usually delivered through red light-emitting diodes attached on goggles which are placed over the patient's closed eyelids [20]. Alternatively, scleral contact lenses may be used [44]. The more typical pattern-reversal stimuli used in clinical settings cannot be used intraoperatively, as they require fixation from an awake patient. Low and high frequency filters are set at 1 and 100 Hz, respectively. The stimulus has a duration of 5 msec and is delivered at rate between 1 and 5 Hz. The analysis time (time base) is set to 300 msec. Approximately 100 single trials are needed for reliable VEP recordings.

7.6.5   *Affecting Factors*

All VEP components are strongly influenced by metabolic factors and changes in anesthesia regime [20].

Nitrous oxide (N_2O) reduces significantly the amplitude of all components but has a small effect on their latency [69].

Inhalational agents, such as *Isoflurane, Halothane,* and *Enflurane,* have the most dramatic effects on VEPs (they drastically decrease the amplitude and increase the latency of the responses [43]) and, thus, they must be completely avoided.

Etomidate slightly increases VEP latencies, and has a small effect on amplitude, especially in combination with other drugs [43].

Diazepam reduces the amplitude, but does not affect the latency of VEPs [43].

Hypothermia below 35°C increases the latency and decreases the amplitude VEPs [69].

7.6.6   VEP Intraoperative Interpretation

In general, after induction and final positioning of the patient, a set of baselines is obtained which remains on the screen for comparison throughout the case. Baseline responses should contain clear and reliable components, and should also be consistent with the clinical picture of the patient.

During surgery, interpretation criteria are based on detection of reliable changes (compared to baselines) that affect the overall morphology of the response, their latency, as well as eventual asymmetry in component amplitude and latency between the left and right eyes [20].

A change can be considered significant if (1) results in a 50% amplitude reduction or complete loss of the VEP, or (2) the maximum latency shift is more than approximately 40–50 msec [69]. However, because of the great variability of the flash VEPs, the only reliable criterion for abnormality is the complete absence of the components resulting from monocular stimulation.

Several studies have shown the high incidence of false positives that can be as high as 95% of the cases, thus making the intraoperative use of VEPs questionable [69].

7.7   Motor Evoked Potentials

7.7.1   Generation

Motor evoked potentials (MEPs) can be generated by electrical or magnetic stimulation of the cortex or the spinal cord [35], however, recent studies have shown that the most reliable ones are those obtained from electrical stimulation of the spinal cord [54]. MEPs can be recorded from either a limb muscle or a peripheral nerve, and the responses obtained are referred to as *myogenic* and *neurogenic* MEPs, respectively.

The organization of the motor system follows closely that of the sensory one. However, in the motor system the flow of activity follows the opposite direction, i.e., from the center to the periphery. Most of the neuronal axons leaving the motor cortex enter the brainstem. There the majority of the fibers decussate and run down the posterolateral section of the spinal cord, whereas the remaining uncrossed fibers run down the anterolateral tracts. Most of the crossed and uncrossed fibers terminate within the spinal cord, where they synapse on an interneuron. The interneuron, in turn, synapses on a motor neuron which is located in the anterior horn of the spinal cord.

Motor neurons innervate skeletal muscles that provide body movement. Figure 7.21 shows a schematic diagram of the motor tract from the cortex to the spinal cord, whereas Figure 7.22 shows the sensory and motor roots at the junction with the spinal cord.

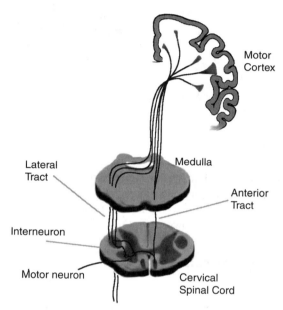

Figure 7.21 Schematic diagram of the motor tract from the cortex to the spinal cord.

7.7.2 Use

Somatosensory EP monitoring measures the integrity of sensory tracts only. Therefore, selective damage to motor tracts may go undetected. Additionally, since the ventral and dorsal portions of the spine are supplied by different blood vessels, ischemia affecting the motor tracts only will not be detected by SEPs. Thus, MEPs are used intraoperatively to protect the structural and functional integrity of the motor tracts in the spinal cord.

7.7.3 MEP Features

Neurogenic MEPs recorded, for example, at the popliteal fossa, in addition to the *orthodromic* motor component, contain an *antidromic* sensory component. The former results from intentional stimulation of the motor tracts in the spinal cord and travels in the direction of normal signal propagation, while the latter results from unintentional stimulation of the sensory tracts in the spinal cord and travels in the

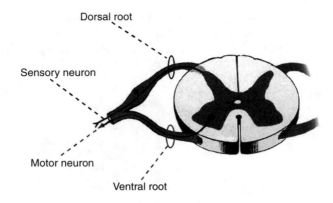

Dorsal root

Sensory neuron

Motor neuron

Ventral root

Figure 7.22   Dorsal and ventral spinal roots and the distribution of the sensory and motor tracts in the spinal cord.

opposite direction of normal signal propagation. However, because of differences in conduction velocity in the sensory and motor tracts, the motor component leads the sensory one, allowing for proper discrimination of the two types of activity [54]. An example of such a recording is shown in Figure 7.23.

7.7.4   Recording Procedure

Stimulation

To elicit MEPs, an electrical stimulus is typically delivered to the spinal cord proximally to the level of surgery. Stimulation can be either *translaminar* or *percutaneous.* In the former case, the stimulating electrodes are placed inside the incision into the base of the spinal processes or, after a laminectomy, into the cancellous bone. In the latter case, electrodes are placed outside the incision, proximal to the surgical field. Electrodes are positioned laterally to the spinous processes, so that their tips lie against the laminae. They should not be placed into the interspinous ligaments. The positive and negative electrodes are placed 2–3 cm apart, usually into adjacent vertebrae [54].

When the surgery involves the high cervical spine, it may not be possible to place two percutaneous electrodes proximal to the incision. In this case, a combination of one percutaneous and one nasopharyngeal electrode may be used.

In general, it is possible to record *myogenic* (activity from muscles) and *neurogenic* (activity from nerves) MEPs.

Myogenic MEPs are obtained with low and high frequency filters set at 10 and 5000 Hz, respectively. Contrary to all recording procedures described so far, the usual stimulus type is constant voltage, with an intensity of about 200 V. The stimulus has a duration of 0.3 msec and is delivered at a rate of 4.7 Hz. The analysis time is set equal to 50 msec. A relatively low sensitivity, between 50 and 100 μV can be used. Typically, no averaging is needed for reliable myogenic MEPs [54].

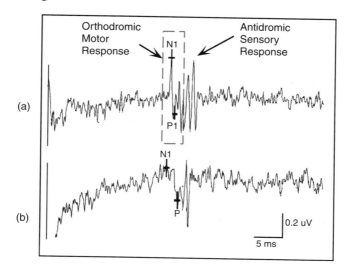

Figure 7.23   Typical MEP recordings obtained from stimulation of the cervical spine showing both the orthodromic (motor) and the antidromic (sensory) components.

Neurogenic MEPs are obtained with slightly different parameters. The low and high frequency filters set at 30 and 2000 Hz, respectively. Again, the stimulus type is constant voltage, with an intensity of up to 300 V. The stimulus has a duration of 0.3 msec and is delivered at a rate of 4.7 Hz. The analysis time is 50 msec. Sensitivity must be as high as possible, typically 1 or 2 μV. Approximately 100 single trials are needed for reliable neurogenic MEPs [54]. The parameters to be used for myogenic and neurogenic MEPs are summarized in Table 7.8.

Table 7.8 Recommended Parameters for Recording Myogenic and Neurogenic MEPs

MEP	Filters	Stimulus Intensity	Stimulus Duration	Stimulus Rate	Sensitivity	Time Base
Myogenic	10–5000 Hz	200 V	0.3 msec	4.7 Hz	50–100 μV	50 msec
Neurogenic	30–2000 Hz	300 V			1–2 μV	

Recording Sites

For myogenic MEPs, electromyographic (EMG) activity is recorded from muscles innervated by the nerve roots at risk, typically from the C_5 to C_7 in the upper body and L_4 to S_1 in the lower body. These muscles are listed in Table 6.4. For neurogenic MEPs, activity is recorded from peripheral nerves in the upper and the lower body, such as the median and the posterior tibial nerves, respectively. Regardless of the type of MEPs studied, all recordings must be bipolar, since the stimulus excites all four limbs of the body simultaneously, thus no quiet site is available to be used as a reference.

7.7.5   Affecting Factors

MEPs are extremely sensitive to anesthetic drugs, especially to inhalational agents, such as nitrous oxide and Isoflurane [28]. Intravenous anesthetics, such as benzo-diazepines, barbiturates, and Propofol, all produce depression of the myogenic and neurogenic MEPs [43].

Anesthesia techniques using a combination of less than 50% nitrous oxide and narcotics, Etomidate, or Ketamine allow the recording of reliable MEPs [28].

The level of muscle relaxation is also critical when recording MEPs. For myogenic MEPs the patient should show 2 out of 4 twitches. If the patient is more relaxed, then MEPs will be degraded or even lost. If the patient is not relaxed, stimulation will produce contraction of the paraspinal muscles, resulting in significant movement of the patient.

For neurogenic MEPs the patient should be completely relaxed, showing 0 out of 4 twitches. Otherwise, the neurogenic and the myogenic responses may overlap, making interpretation extremely difficult [54].

7.7.6   MEP Intraoperative Interpretation

While the latency of myogenic MEPs is very consistent, their morphology and am-plitude can vary wildly. Therefore, intraoperative interpretation is based only on the presence or absence of a response. On the other hand, neurogenic MEPs show more reliable morphology, amplitude, and latency. However, the most sensitive criterion for intraoperative interpretation is based only on amplitude. A 60% amplitude reduc-tion is considered a strong indication to warn the surgeon, whereas 80% reduction qualifies as a reliable change that requires intervention [54].

7.8   Triggered EMG

7.8.1   Generation

Triggered electromyographic (tEMG) activity can be recorded from a muscle after di-rect electrical stimulation of the motor nerve or nerve root that innervates that muscle. These signals are also known as compound muscle action potentials (CMAPs).

7.8.2   Use

Intraoperatively tEMG is used in several types of neurological and orthopedic surgery that involve the brain or the spinal cord. For example, during posterior fossa surgery for acoustic tumor or lumbosacral spinal canal surgery for tethered cord, nerves or nerve roots may not be visible in the surgical field due to anatomical deformations.

The use of direct stimulation can verify the presence of healthy neural tissue and its functionality.

Also, during placement of spinal instrumentation, a misplaced pedicle screw that has fractured the bone and, thus, is threatening a rootlet can be detected by stimulating the screw and determining the current threshold necessary to elicit a response in a muscle innervated by that rootlet [7]. In general, tEMG is used to:

- Identify specific cranial nerves or nerve roots.

- Protect structural and functional integrity of cranial nerves and spinal nerve roots.

- Identify neural tissue embedded in a tumor or lipoma.

- Verify functional integrity of neural tissue and make decisions on aggressiveness of procedure.

- Verify structural integrity of pedicles.

- Verify placement of pedicle screws.

7.8.3   *tEMG Features*

Similarly to spontaneous EMG (see Section 6.3), intraoperative tEMG interpretation is based on the presence or absence of a response. In some cases, however, the latency of the response may be important in determining the identity of the stimulated nerve. For example, when the V and the VII cranial nerves are stimulated simultaneously, the response from the V nerve leads the one from the VII nerve by approximately 2 msec [48].

7.8.4   *Recording Procedure*

Stimulation

Depending on the surgical procedure, stimulation can be monopolar or bipolar. Monopolar stimulation is delivered with a hand-held single-tip stimulator, which is used as the cathode (negative stimulating electrode). The anode (positive electrode) consists of a sterile subdermal needle placed into a muscle inside the incision. Bipolar stimulation is delivered with a double tip electrode, with the negative tip placed towards the recording site.

Constant-current stimuli, each having a duration of 0.01 msec, are delivered at a low rate of 1 or 2 Hz to avoid muscle fatigue. Stimulus intensity for direct nerve or nerve root stimulation is gradually increased from 0 mA until an EMG response is seen, up to a maximum of about 2 mA [48]. For pedicle or pedicle screw stimulation, stimulus intensity is gradually increased until a response is seen, from 0 mA up to a maximum of approximately 40 mA [7, 54]. This procedure is used to minimize the amount of current delivered to neural structures.

Recording Sites

Placement of the recording electrodes, the selection muscles for recording, and recording parameters have been described in Section 6.3. Besides having the EMG signal displayed on the computer screen for proper latency determination, it is advantageous to present it through a loudspeaker, so that the surgical team can hear any muscle activity [44].

7.8.5   Affecting Factors

As in the case of spontaneous EMG, the most important factor is muscle relaxation. For proper monitoring the patient should be reversed or slightly relaxed, showing three twitches out of a train of four [44, 57].

7.8.6   tEMG Intraoperative Interpretation

Direct stimulation of a nerve or nerve root will result in activity in a muscle innervated by it. Interpretation of the response obtained depends on the procedure being monitored as it is indicated below:

Identification of Cranial Nerves

By simply determining the muscle on which a response has been obtained one can resolve the identity of the cranial nerve under test. If the same recording electrode detects activity from a muscle corresponding to two different nerves (as in the case of an electrode on the masseter which may detect responses from both the V and the VII cranial nerves) then the latency of the response will determine its origin [48].

Identification of Root Level

Since the same rootlet innervates several muscles, interpretation criteria for identification of the nerve root when multiple muscles are monitored simultaneously are based on correlating the pattern of activity observed with muscles that respond and muscles that do not [54, 57].

Identification of Neural Tissue

Often healthy neural tissue is embedded in a tumor or lipoma. After stimulation of different parts of the tissue, only those fibers producing a response correspond to functional neural tissue and, thus, need to be preserved.

Pedicle Screw Placement

Verification of pedicle integrity during placement of pedicle screws is common in those procedures involving instrumentation. Sequential stimulation of the intact pedicle, tapped pedicle, pedicle hole, and pedicle screw at the same root level will determine various current thresholds necessary to elicit a response. A drastic difference among these thresholds is indicative of a screw misplacement (the screw may have cracked the bone and entered into the vicinity of the rootlet) [7].

The threshold necessary to elicit a response using constant current stimulation of the intact pedicle varies among subjects, but a typical value is around 40 mA [7].

Placement of a screw may slightly decrease this threshold, without any damage to the bone. However, a threshold to screw stimulation of less than about 10 mA is typically an indication of a misplacement [7].

7.9 *Review Questions*

1. What do ERs represent?

2. Explain the rationale for using ERs intraoperatively.

3. What are the two main categories of ERs?

4. Are ERs and EPs the same?

5. What is the difference between sensory and motor EPs?

6. When are baseline EPs collected?

7. How are SEPs generated?

8. Describe the main pathway between the stimulation and the recording sites in median nerve SEPs.

9. Describe the main pathway between the stimulation and the recording sites in tibial nerve SEPs.

10. What is the use of SEPs intraoperatively?

11. How many recording sites do SEP monitoring protocols usually include? Which ones?

12. How similar, in terms of amplitude and latency, should repeated SEPs from stimulation of the same limbs be?

13. What is the maximum amplitude and latency difference between the SEPs obtained from the two arms or legs?

14. What are the stimulation and recording parameter for median nerve SEPs?

15. What are the stimulation and recording parameter for tibial nerve SEPs?

16. What are the latencies of the three main components obtained in median nerve SEPs?

17. What are the latencies of the three main components obtained in tibial nerve SEPs?

18. Describe the effect that anesthetic agents have on the cortical and subcortical SEP components.

19. What are the effects of hypotension on cortical and subcortical SEP components?

20. What are the criteria for determining whether an SEP amplitude or latency change is reliable?

21. What are the criteria for determining whether an SEP amplitude or latency change is significant?

22. How do changes due to perisurgical factors differ from changes due to surgical intervention?

23. What are the dermatomes?

24. How are DSEPs obtained?

25. What is the intraoperative use of DSEPs?

26. Explain why SEP monitoring is not root specific.

27. What kind of responses is it easier to obtain, SEPs or DSEPs? Explain why.

28. What parameters can be used for recording DSEPs?

29. Do DSEPs corresponding to different spinal levels have the same latency?

30. What is the most important feature for interpreting DSEPs?

31. What are the generators of BAERs?

32. Describe the approximate morphology of the first 10 msec of a BAER?

33. What brain structure is responsible for the generation of peak V?

34. What are the three most reliable peaks in a BAER?

35. How can the amplitude of BAER peak I be improved?

36. What is the main difference between an ipsilateral and a contralateral BAER?

37. Give the montage used for recording BAERs?

38. Give the parameters used for recording BAERs?

39. When recording BAERs, are both ears stimulated simultaneously? Explain.

40. What is the role of noise delivered to the contralateral ear during stimulation of the ipsilateral ear?

41. Describe the effect of nitrous oxide on BAERs.

42. What is more likely to be affected by intravenous anesthetics, the amplitude or the latency of a BAER?

43. State the criteria used for interpreting intraoperative BAERs.

44. What are the generators of VEPs.

45. What is the primary intraoperative use of VEPs?

46. Describe the main VEP components and their latencies.

47. What kind of montage is used for recording VEPs?

48. What kind of visual stimuli are used to elicit intraoperative VEPs?

49. Are VEPs relatively resistant to anesthetic agents?

50. What criteria are used for identifying significant VEP changes?

51. Overall, are intraoperative VEPs reliable?

52. How are MEPs elicited?

53. Describe the two categories of MEPs.

54. Describe the gross anatomy of the motor and sensory tracts in the spinal cord.

55. Why are MEPs needed?

56. After electrical stimulation of the spinal cord at the neck, what kind of responses can be recorded at the popliteal fossa?

57. How can one differentiate an orthodromic motor from an antidromic sensory response?

58. What parameters are used for recording myogenic MEPs?

59. What parameters are used for recording neurogenic MEPs?

60. Is it necessary to use bipolar recordings to record MEPs? Explain.

61. Are MEPs sensitive to anesthetic agents?

62. What kind of muscle relaxation is needed to record myogenic MEPs?

63. What kind of muscle relaxation is needed to record neurogenic MEPs?

64. How is tEMG generated?

65. What are the uses of tEMG?

66. Give the interpretation criteria for tEMG.

67. Give the parameters recommended for direct nerve root stimulation.

68. Describe the procedure for verification of appropriate placement of pedicle screws.

69. Give the parameters recommended for stimulation of pedicle screws.

chapter 8

Spine Surgery

8.1   Introduction

The *vertebral column,* or backbone, is divided into five regions, namely *cervical, thoracic, lumbar, sacral,* and *coccygeal* [74], as is schematically shown in Figure 8.1. There are 24 individual bony segments, known as *vertebrae,* in addition to the sacral and coccygeal ones that are fused. Each vertebra consists of an anterior body and

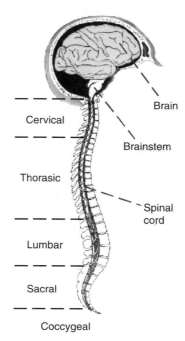

Figure 8.1   Schematic diagram of a vertebral column showing its various regions.

a posterior arch that enclose the *vertebral foramen*. The *spinal cord* lies within the *spinal canal*, which is formed by the foramina of the vertebrae. Such an arrangement is shown in Figure 8.2.

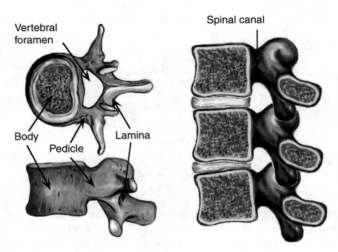

Figure 8.2   Schematic diagram of a vertebra.

A large number of neurosurgical procedures involve the spinal column and the spinal cord. However, the common objective in most cases is the correction of deformity, stabilization of unstable spinal levels, decompression of neural tissue, or a combination of the above [17].

Spinal deformities do not always require surgery. Indeed, intervention is indicated only when it is accompanied by pain, when its progression may result in neurologic or pulmonary dysfunction, or for cosmetic reasons. The procedure requires the use of spinal instrumentation (permanent metallic implants) and it is supplemented by *fusion*, i.e., bridging of one vertebra to another through solid bone. Fusion is almost always needed, since continued stress on metallic implants can cause them to fail [11].

Stabilization of the spine is needed whenever motion of certain spinal levels that have become unstable, or changes in some intervertebral disc or facet joints, are accompanied by pain and there is also the potential risk for neurologic injury. In those cases, surgical intervention involves the elimination of motion through rigid implants and spinal fusion.

Decompression entails the removal of any material, such as disk, bone, or tumor, that places undue pressure on neural tissue, including the spinal cord, spinal roots, conus medullaris, and cauda equina, which are schematically shown in Figure 8.3. Finally, surgery may involve the spine itself, for instance, in the case of a spinal tumor or the spinal roots. The latter is true, for example, in the management of spasticity which, as explained in Section 8.8, requires selective rhizotomy [67]).

Depending upon the particular characteristics of each case, the surgeon may choose to follow an *anterior, posterior,* or *combined* anteroposterior approach.[1] However, the most common technique is directly posterior, which allows exposure of the spinous processes, laminae, and facet joints of the entire spine [17]. In general, the posterior approach is associated with lower risks than the anterior one.

Like every other surgical procedure, a neurosurgical operation entails risks for events that are both unwanted and unplanned. In general, complications can be classified into two major categories: those associated with a significant reduction in the blood supply in a particular region of the central nervous system, a condition known as *ischemia,* and those associated with *mechanical injury* of neural tissue. Fortunately, in most cases both types of complications can be, and they are, avoided. Intraoperative electrophysiological monitoring (IOM) has been proven very useful in reducing some long-term complications of neurosurgical intervention, because it provides on-line measures of the functional integrity of the nervous system [28, 44, 54]. The most common procedures of spinal surgery along with the associated risks and the specific neurophysiological tests that may help reduce these risks are summarized in Table 8.1.

The most widely employed approach to monitoring the functional integrity of the spinal cord consists of recording somatosensory evoked potentials (SEPs) in response to electrical stimulation of either the posterior tibial nerve at the ankle, or the median nerve at the wrist [11, 44, 57, 77]. These procedures are described in detail in Sections 7.3.5 and 7.3.6, respectively.

However, one should be aware that SEPs reflect neural activity predominantly in the *dorsal* (posterior) columns of the spinal cord which consist of mainly ascending *somatosensory* pathways. Although surgical insults to the *ventral* (anterior) parts of the cord, which include the descending *motor* pathways, are very likely to interfere with the function of the somatosensory pathways as well, there is evidence suggesting that the ascending sensory and the descending motor pathways differ in their susceptibility to external trauma. The functional integrity of the motor pathways can be assessed reliably using motor evoked potentials (MEPs) elicited by electrical stimulation of the spinal cord. The stimulation site is proximal while the recording site is distal to the level of the surgery [57]. A detailed description of this procedure is given in Section 7.7.

The *conus medullaris* is a tapering of the *lumbar enlargement* at the lower extremity of the spinal cord and marks the beginning of the *cauda equina,* which is a bundle of spinal nerve roots arising from this area, as it is schematically shown in Figure 8.3.

When surgery is below the conus medullaris, the integrity of individual nerve roots during tissue exploration or placement of instrumentation can be monitored by recording spontaneous or triggered electromyographic (EMG) activity from the muscles innervated by the nerve roots at risk. Details about these procedures are

[1]Less often surgery follows a *transoral* approach, i.e., through an incision in the back of the mouth. This procedure is reserved for the treatment of abnormalities involving the cervical vertebrae Ci and Cii, which are also known as the *atlas* and the *odontoid* bones, respectively.

Table 8.1 Examples of Surgical Procedures Involving the Spine, Associated Risks, and Neurophysiological Tests Administered to Minimize These Risks

Procedure	Risks	Tests Administered
Scoliosis, kyphosis	Spinal cord injury during distraction; ischemia due to artery occlusion.	Post. tibial n. SEPs, MEPs.
Spondylolisthesis, fractures, stenosis	Spinal cord and root injury during manipulation; cord or leg ischemia due to artery occlusion; root damage during pedicle screw placement.	Post. tibial n. SEPs, MEPs, EMG, tEMG.
Disc disease	Spinal cord and root injury during discectomy and interbody fusion; ischemia.	Median (c_1–c_6), Ulnar (c_7), tibial SEPs (c_7–L_5), MEPs, EMG, tEMG.
Tumors	Spinal cord and root injury during resection; ischemia.	Median (c_1–c_6), Ulnar (c_7), tibial SEPs (c_7–L_5), MEPs, EMG, tEMG.
Aneurysms, AVMs	Spinal cord, leg and brain ischemia.	Tibial n. SEPs, MEPs, EEG.
Tethered cord	Nerve root injury.	EMG, tEMG
Dorsal rhizotomy	Nerve root injury.	tEMG

given in Sections 6.3 and 7.8. Alternative techniques involving dermatomal SEPs (DSEPs) have also been proposed [71] and they are described in Section 7.4.

Finally, proper positioning of the patient on the surgical table is extremely important. Excessive traction and pressure on sensitive areas, such as the brachial plexus and the ulnar nerve, must be avoided. To monitor brachial plexus function and avoid possible brachial plexopathy it is recommended that, in addition to any other test administered, SEPs to ulnar nerve stimulation be monitored, at least occasionally, especially in cases whereby one may think that only SEPs to posterior tibial nerve would be enough [54].

The above-mentioned standard neurophysiological techniques for monitoring the spine, along with their technical details and possible interpretation of the results obtained intraoperatively, are explained in detail in previous chapters. In this chapter, we give some specific examples of spinal surgery where intraoperative monitoring has been shown to be of great help to the surgeons, especially during critical phases of the procedures.

8.2   Spinal Deformities

Surgery in the spinal column is often necessary for the correction of spinal deformities, the most common types of which are scoliosis and kyphosis (hunchback). *Scoliosis*

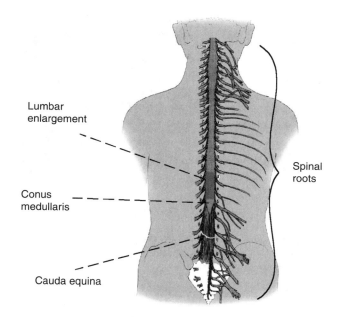

Lumbar
enlargement

Spinal
roots

Conus
medullaris

Cauda equina

Figure 8.3   Schematic diagram of the various structures found in the lower extremity of the spinal cord.

is characterized by a lateral curvature of the spine which is accompanied by rotation of the vertebrae toward the concavity of the curve. *Kyphosis,* on the other hand, is an abnormal posterior deviation of the spine usually in the thoracic and lumbar levels. A schematic diagram of one possibility of lateral curvature in a scoliotic spine is seen in Figure 8.4(a).

Surgical management of scoliosis has two objectives: (1) to partially correct the deformity using metal implants, and (2) to permanently stabilize the excessively curved area of the spine through bony fusion [17]. Depending on the age of the patient and the etiology of the disease, surgery may involve partial anterior or posterior spinal fusion with instrumentation. The first successful and most widely used approach to the surgical management of scoliosis involves an inflexible metal rod, as shown in Figure 8.4(b). This device, known as the *Harrington rod,* is attached to the side of the thoracolumbar spine with the aid of hooks, as shown in Figure 8.4(c).

Another technique, known as *segmental fixation,* stabilizes multiple individual vertebrae throughout the curve [17]. A combination of hooks, screws, and wires may be used. After rod placement, the spine is distracted to reduce the concavity of the curve, fused with bone graft taken previously from the exposed vertebrae, and kept in its new position with the rods. An alternative technique involves the insertion of a wire under the vertebral laminae above and below the concavity, which is then stretched to straighten the spine. Surgical management for kyphosis is similar to that

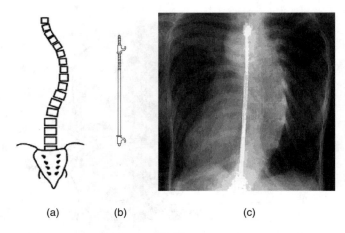

(a)   (b)   (c)

Figure 8.4   Example of scoliosis. (a) Schematic diagram of the lateral curvature of the spine and (b) the Harrington rod used to correct (c) the deformity.

used for scoliosis. A typical case entails anterior fusion, and posterior fusion with instrumentation [1].

The most feared complication of these procedures is damage to the spinal cord, and the surgical manipulations that are associated with the greatest risk are distraction and derotation of the vertebrae. Excessive maneuvering can cause mechanical injury, stretching and compression of the spinal cord, or occlusion of blood vessels that supply the cord. Unwanted neurological complications, such as loss of leg strength, have been reported to occur in as many as 1 to 2% of the cases [37].

The procedure of choice for monitoring the functional integrity of the spinal cord is the recording of SEPs in response to electrical stimulation of the posterior tibial nerve at the ankle [7, 18], as described in Section 7.3.6. Stimulation is applied distal and recorded both distal and proximal to the surgical levels. In addition, the functional integrity of the motor pathway specifically can be assessed using MEPs elicited by electrical stimulation of the spinal cord, as described in Section 7.7.4. In this case, stimulation is applied proximal and recorded distal to the level of the surgery. The exact procedures for recording and interpreting the results thus obtained can be found in Chapter 7.

Briefly, monitoring focuses on the amplitude and latency of the cervical and cortical responses, looking for even small changes during or immediately after a specific maneuver, e.g., distraction. Often, however, the parameters of the cortical responses display a great deal of variability during the surgical procedure, because they are highly susceptible to perisurgical factors and especially anesthesia. In these cases, the parameters of the cervical responses become the primary focus of monitoring.

To monitor brachial plexus function and avoid possible brachial plexopathy from improper positioning of a patient's shoulders on the surgical table, it is recommended that SEPs to ulnar nerve stimulation be monitored as well [54], as described in Section 8.9.3.

8.3   Disc Disease

Intervertebral disks are composite structures that link adjacent vertebrae while allowing multiplanar motion. Each disk is composed of two main parts, the *annulus* and
the *nucleus,* which correspond to the outer part and the more gelatinous inner area,
respectively. *Disc herniation* occurs when some of the annular fibers are disrupted
and the nuclear material is displaced [17]. Depending on the degree of herniation,
the displaced material may cause a bulging of the outermost annular fibers or, in the
worst case, it may enter the spinal canal as a free fragment.

A schematic diagram of a herniated disc along with and an MRI picture are shown
in Figure 8.5(a) and Figure 8.5(b), respectively, where a bulged disc has entered the
spinal canal and is pressing on the spinal cord.

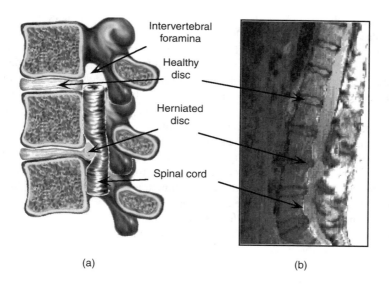

(a)   (b)

Figure 8.5   (a) Drawing and (b) MRI picture of a herniated disc that has entered the spinal
canal and is pressing on the spinal cord.

Disc herniation can occur at any level of the spine, but the thoracic discs are less
frequently affected than the lumbar or the cervical ones [17]. It is estimated [74] that
approximately 1 to 2% of the general population will experience leg pain caused by
a herniated lumbar disc that compresses one or more nerve roots (a condition also
known as *radiculopathy*) or constricts the spinal canal (resulting in what is known
as *spinal stenosis*). Surgical intervention may cause injury to the spinal cord at the
time of removal of the damaged disc (a procedure referred to as *discectomy*) and the
insertion of bone graft in place of the removed disk. Additionally, during placement
of instrumentation, inappropriate placement of pedicle screws may damage individual
roots. It should be kept in mind that the risk for neural injury to the cord and possibly
to the nerve roots is higher when myelopathy is a preexisting condition.

Surgery for disc disease can be performed following an anterior or a posterior approach [11]. In many cases an anterior procedure is indicated instead of, or in addition to, the posterior one. In cervical spine cases, the anterior approach is often preferred when discectomy followed by interbody fusion is necessary. The anterior approach is associated with the additional risk for vascular complications (e.g., ischemia), due to the close proximity of the areas of interest to major blood vessels, such as the carotid, the vertebral, and the anterior spinal arteries in the cervical area, or the iliac artery in the lumbar region [59]. Arterial injury or unplanned occlusion may have devastating consequences for the functional integrity of the spinal cord. For example, unnoticed placement of a retractor on the anterior spinal artery can cause severe ischemia due to the lack of sufficient collateral blood flow. Such an event can occur virtually at any time during the procedure, even before any direct surgical manipulation of the spine has been initiated.

In general, the incidence of postoperative neurological complications associated with these surgical procedures, although not very high, are certainly not negligible (estimates for the posterior and the anterior approach run in the order of 0.64 and 2.18%, respectively [74]), thus rendering the routine use of IOM highly desirable. Continuous recording of SEPs is the standard monitoring technique. Median nerve stimulation should be used for operations above the level of the sixth vertebra (Cvi). If the Cvii level is also involved ulnar nerve stimulation is preferable. Finally, for operations below the Cvii SEPs to posterior tibial nerve stimulation are indicated.

When monitoring SEPs, both the amplitude and latency of the cervical component should be closely followed throughout the case [54]. In most instances, also the cortical component can be recorded consistently throughout the procedure, and it can serve as an additional measure of the functional integrity of the spinal cord. Interpretation criteria are described in Chapters 6 and 7.

It is not uncommon, however, to observe variations in the latency of the cervical component during the procedure that are due to systemic factors, such as hypothermia or hypotension. In these cases the latency of the peripheral response is also prolonged. The SEP response recorded over the cervical spine following stimulation at the wrist is perhaps the most sensitive indication of cord damage. When monitoring median nerve SEPs, a useful strategy that can help avoid raising unnecessary concerns is to monitor, from the beginning of the procedure, the delay between the peripheral response (recorded at Erb's point) and the cervical component. This latency difference, which normally is around 4 msec, is affected to a lesser degree by perisurgical factors than the absolute latency of the cervical response per se.

Occasionally, and especially during anterior procedures in the lumbosacral spine, the surgeon may intentionally place a vascular clip in one of the iliac arteries. In these cases, the intraoperative monitoring personnel should be able to localize such an ischemic insult and, when interpreting the changes detected, they should be able to differentiate intentional from unintentional ischemia.

For example, temporary occlusion of vessels that feed the cervical spinal cord would lead to a deterioration of the cervical *and* cortical SEP components elicited by stimulation of the posterior tibial nerve of the *ipsilateral* leg [59]. However, the responses recorded at the popliteal fossa (behind the knee) would remain unaffected.

On the other hand, temporary occlusion of the abdominal aorta, or one of the vessels that supply the legs such as, for instance, the iliac artery, would cause a partial or complete loss of all responses (including the peripheral ones) *ipsilateral* to the side of the occluded artery. An example of this last situation is shown in Figure 8.6 where an inadvertent occlusion of the left iliac artery was detected. Notice the increase in latency and decrease in amplitude of all responses to left-leg stimulation shown in Figure 8.6(a), while the responses to right-leg stimulation shown in Figure 8.6(b) are unaffected. All changes are computed with reference to the baselines, shown in a lighter color in the figure, which are collected at the beginning of the operation.

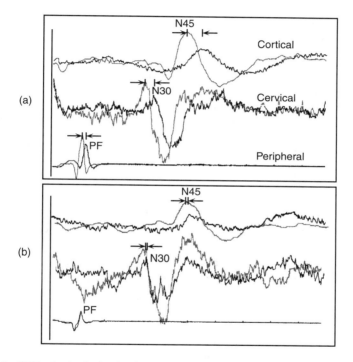

Figure 8.6   SEPs obtained after inadvertent occlusion of the left iliac artery. (a) Increased latency and decreased amplitude is seen in all responses to left-leg stimulation, while (b) the responses to right-leg stimulation remain unaffected. Light-color traces correspond to the baselines collected at the beginning of the operation.

After reversal of the insult that caused ischemia, and especially in cases of intentional vessel occlusion, all responses should fully recover within 15 to 20 min. In this case, the amplitude of the peripheral response can be used as an index of adequate perfusion after the clip has been removed.

In the cervical area, accidental occlusion of the carotid artery during an anterior approach may cause cortical ischemia. In that case, the parameters of the cortical responses can be used as indices of brain perfusion. Deterioration of the cortical response recorded in the hemisphere *contralateral* to the side of the operation that is accompanied by a prolongation of the cervical-cortical interpeak delay,[2] while the cervical response remains unaffected, may be indicative of a vascular insult to the carotid artery (most probably the result of a misplaced retractor).

In some cases, MEPs may be more sensitive indices of spinal cord damage because it is the anterior part of the cord that is more directly affected by a herniated disc. Finally, we recommend monitoring of EMG during root manipulation and tEMG during pedicle screw placement. These procedures are described in Section 7.7. The functional integrity of individual roots can also be assessed using DSEPs [71] which are described in Section 7.4.

8.4   *Spinal Fractures and Instabilities*

Several conditions may affect the normal structure, function, and stability of the spine. These include degenerative diseases such as *rheumatoid arthritis, spondylosis, spondylitis,* and *stenosis,* as well as, spondylolisthesis and fractures. The affected areas may involve the intervertebral discs, the facet joints, or the vertebral bone, causing a distortion of the spinal anatomy and posing a direct threat to the spine and the spinal roots. Depending on the particular case and its severity, patients may experience no symptoms at all, or they may develop symptoms, ranging from local discomfort to pain and weakness in their extremities. Neurological deterioration following these procedures has been reported to occur in approximately 1% of the cases [2].

Degenerative conditions often necessitate surgical intervention in order to stabilize the spine and reduce the neurological deficits, or simply to arrest the progression of symptoms.

In *spinal fractures,* on the other hand, compression or damage of the cord by bone and disc fragments that enter the spinal canal is a common threat. Surgical management of these cases requires fusion with instrumentation whereby metal rods are used to stabilize the spine. In addition, it may be necessary to decompress the cord and restore the volume of the spinal canal. A schematic diagram of a fractured vertebra is shown in Figure 8.7, while MRI examples of spinal fractures in the cervical and thoracic areas are shown in Figure 8.8.

Figure 8.9 shows a schematic diagram of a plating system used to correct spinal fractures. A different type of implantable system is shown in Figure 8.10(a), where part of the various implants are shown. Figure 8.10(b) shows the procedure for tapping a spinal pedicle, while the final assembly of instrumentation is depicted in Figure 8.10(c).

Spondylolisthesis typically occurs in the lumbar spine and it is manifested by a horizontal displacement of one vertebra over another. An example of this condition is shown in Figure 8.11. The procedure of choice for reduction of the abnormal

---

[2]This measure is known as *central conduction time.*

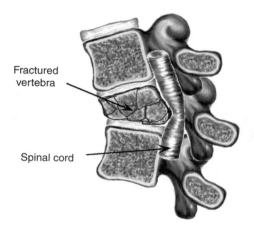

Figure 8.7   Schematic diagram of a fractured vertebra with fragments pressing on the spinal cord.

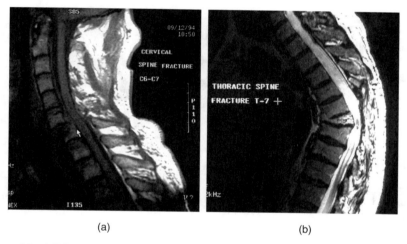

(a)   (b)

Figure 8.8   MRI examples of spinal fractures in the (a) cervical and (b) thoracic areas.

vertebral displacement is fusion with internal fixation using a metal plate held in place with pedicle screws.

A variety of complications can occur during these operations, most of which are common to all spine surgeries, regardless of whether the surgeon follows an anterior, posterior, or combined anteroposterior approach [11]. The primary risks include: (1) direct mechanical insult to the spinal cord and to the nerve roots, due to the placement of the instrumentation; (2) compression or stretching of the cord, due to overdistraction; and (3) vascular insult. The latter is most often seen in anterior approaches to decompression.

An example of detection of cord injury due to misplaced instrumentation is shown in Figure 8.12. The baseline SEPs obtained at the beginning of the case are shown

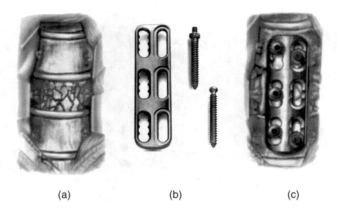

(a)   (b)   (c)

Figure 8.9   Schematic diagram of (a) a fractured vertebra and the plating system (b) before, and (c) after implantation.

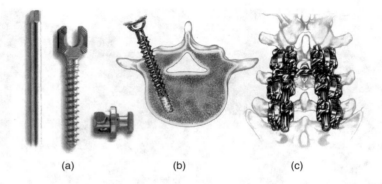

(a)   (b)   (c)

Figure 8.10   Schematic diagram of a pedicle screw spinal system. (a) Part of the implants, (b) the tapped pedicle, and (c) the system in place.

in Figure 8.12(a) along with the time of the recording. Small but normal amplitude and latency variations are recorded throughout the case as shown in Figure 8.12(b). However, just after placement of instrumentation, both the cortical (peak N45) and cervical (peak N30) responses disappear, as shown in Figure 8.12(c), while the peripheral response (peak PF) obtained from the popliteal fossa remain unchanged.

Recording of SEPs is the most widely used monitoring technique. SEPs can be supplemented by MEPs especially when there is a preexisting compression of the anterior part of the cord by bone fragments from the vertebral body. It should be noted that not all spinal fracture cases can be monitored electrophysiologically since, sometimes, the damage to the spinal cord is severe enough to cause temporary or permanent disruption of its function. In such cases, SEPs cannot be recorded consistently and thus they cannot provide adequate intraoperative information.

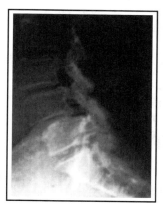

Figure 8.11 MRI example of spondylolisthesis in the lumbar area.

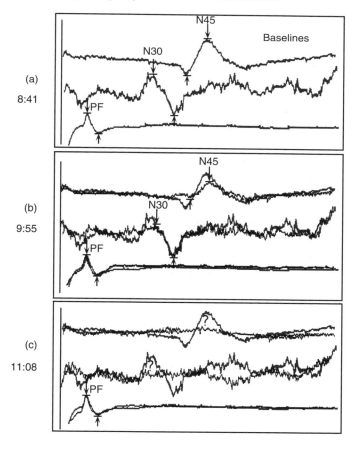

Figure 8.12 SEP recordings obtained after cord injury due to misplaced instrumentation; (a) baselines; (b) normal variations during the case; and (c) cortical (peak N45) and cervical response (peak N30) disappear just after placement of instrumentation, while the peripheral response (peak PF) remains unchanged.

8.5   Tumors

Surgery of the spine is often necessary for the management of tumors. Those that cause neurological symptoms by compressing nerve roots or constricting the spinal canal are known as *extramedullary tumors*. Less frequently tumors grow inside the spinal cord and they are referred to as *intramedullary*. In both cases, however, surgery for tumor removal is performed inside the spinal canal and entails stabilization of the spine with wires or a plate system. Consequently, these procedures are associated with a relatively high incidence of neurological complications, which includes vascular insults (caused by damage or inadvertent occlusion of a major blood vessel) and direct injury to functionally intact neural tissue adjacent to the tumor to be resected.

Intraoperative monitoring typically involves recordings of SEPs. Monitoring of MEPs may also be beneficial, especially when the tumor is located anteriorly and puts the anterior part of the spinal cord at risk. In these cases, the anterior spinal arteries are also at risk, especially during the phases of tissue exploration and tumor removal.

As mentioned previously, monitoring of upper extremity cortical SEPs is highly recommended as a means for detecting vascular insults involving the carotid and the vertebral arteries. Remember that a change in the contralateral cortical response (manifested as a change in amplitude with or without a change in latency) while the cervical response remains unaffected *may* indicate the presence of ischemia developing between the lower brainstem and the cerebral cortex. Such a condition may be caused by accidental occlusion of the vertebral or the carotid artery, most likely by a misplaced retractor.

8.6   Vascular Abnormalities

A schematic diagram of the vascular supply in the thoraco-abdominal areas of the spinal cord is shown in Figure 8.13. Surgery in those areas is often required to repair some vascular abnormality, the most common of which is *abdominal aortic aneurysm*

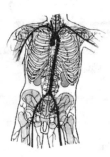

Figure 8.13   Schematic diagram of the vascular supply to the spinal cord in the thoraco-abdominal area.

(AAA). An *aneurysm* is an abnormal dilation (ballooning) of an artery that presents the potential risk of rupture and clotting. The size of an aneurysm varies from a few millimeters to several centimeters. Those over 2.5 cm are termed *giant* aneurysms. Figure 8.14(a) shows an image of the normal aorta, while Figure 8.14(b) shows an example of an aortic aneurysm. Usually aneurysms in the abdomen remain silent until a medical emergency occurs. Rupture of an AAA often causes an irreversible hemorrhagic shock, leading to death.

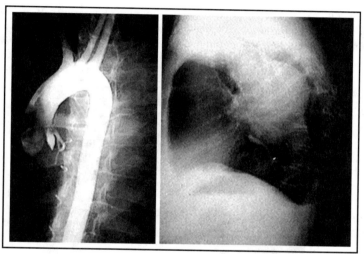

Figure 8.14   (a) Normal aorta and (b) example of aortic aneurysm.

Similarly, *arteriovenous malformations* (AVMs) are abnormal communications between arteries and veins whereby blood is shunted directly from the arterial system to the venous system. An AVM alters the flow of blood supply to the spinal cord by "stealing" blood from surrounding tissues. This can result in ischemia (poor oxygen delivery) and possibly infarction (death of the tissues).

Surgery often involves cross-clamping of the aorta, which is a major source of blood supply to the spinal cord and to the nerves of the lower extremities, among other structures. In these cases, monitoring of lower extremity SEPs and MEPs is used to provide information about the status of the cord which is at risk even when a femoral bypass has been placed. If aortic clamping leads to deep and prolonged ischemia, it can cause permanent damage to the spinal cord and paraplegia.

In almost all cases of aortic cross-clamping, a loss of SEP responses will occur eventually. It is generally accepted that the rate at which SEP parameters change, and the duration of SEP deterioration, are the most reliable predictors of postoperative neurological deficit. Loss of SEP responses within the first five minutes after cross-clamping is a sign of severe ischemia and should be taken as a serious warning for imminent neurological damage. The prognosis appears to be more favorable if the SEP changes are first noticed at least 15 to 20 min after clamping.

Finally, like the previous procedures, monitoring of the brachial plexus function is necessary via ulnar nerve SEPs.

8.7   Tethered Cord

Surgery is often required for the management of malformations in the lumbosacral spine, such as lipomeningocele, myelomeningocele, and diastematomyelia. Figure 8.15 shows an example of a mass in the lower spinal cord that requires surgical intervention. One of the most common sequelae of these conditions is *tethered cord,*

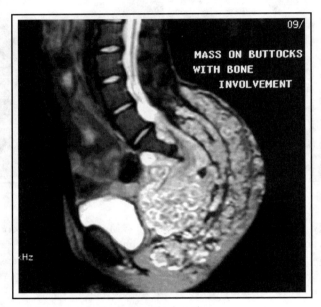

Figure 8.15   Example of mass in the lower spinal cord.

which is characterized by the pathological fixation of the spinal cord in an abnormal caudal location. As the spinal canal grows, the nerve roots in the cauda equina become stretched leading to a number of progressive neurological symptoms. An example of tethered cord is shown in Figure 8.16. In addition to the pediatric population, tethered cord is occasionally seen in adults secondary to the growth of mass lesions in the lower lumbar region and cauda equina.

During operations for tethered cord release, the presence of lipomatous and fibro-matous tissue in the spinal canal renders the identification of functional neural tissue particularly difficult. Nerve roots in the cauda equina often become encased within the abnormal tissue and cannot be easily visualized. The surgeon is primarily inter-

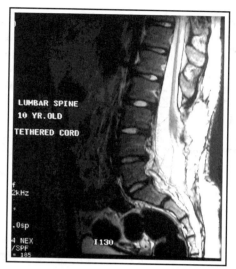

Figure 8.16   Example of tethered cord in a pediatric patient.

ested in identifying the exact location of a nerve root and verifying that it remains functionally intact throughout the procedure.

To fulfill these requirements, electrophysiological monitoring should involve the recording of both spontaneous and triggered EMG from muscles determined by the location of the deformity and the nerve roots at risk. As shown in Table 6.4, bilateral recordings from three sets of muscles, namely the rectus femoris, tibialis anterior, and gastrocnemius, are sufficient to cover levels L_2 to S_1, whereas a pair of EMG electrodes inserted into the anal sphincter should be used if the S_2 to S_4 levels are also at risk. Electrophysiological monitoring of the external anal sphincter is particularly effective in helping preserve the function of both the anal and the urethral sphincters. Spontaneous EMG should be recorded continuously during the procedure in order to detect responses that are indicative of nerve irritation.

8.8   *Selective Dorsal Rhizotomy*

Spasticity is manifested by increased resistance to passive movement, abnormally increased muscle reflexes, and involuntary spasms of muscle contractions. Spasticity in children is one of the manifestations of cerebral palsy caused by a brain insult in the perinatal period. The lesion disrupts the inhibitory action of descending corticospinal inputs on the large spinal motor neurons located in the anterior horn of the spinal cord. Normally, afferent (i.e., sensory) inputs from specialized muscle receptors enter the spinal cord via the dorsal roots and exert an excitatory influence on neurons in the anterior horn. In turn, these spinal motor neurons control muscle tension (spinal reflex arc). The role of the corticospinal inputs is to regulate the net output of the spinal reflex arc so that the tone in each muscle is maintained at a level that is appropriate for the intended posture or movement. In cerebral palsy, damage to the corticospinal inputs leaves the action of the spinal motor neurons unopposed, leading to an overall increase in muscle tone.

One way to control spasticity is to selectively resect the dorsal sensory roots [67], a procedure known as *rhizotomy,* in order to reduce the abnormal excitatory input on anterior horn cells. Indiscriminate resection of dorsal roots would result in complete sensory loss. Triggered EMG recorded intraoperatively from leg muscles and elicited by direct electrical stimulation of individual rootlets can be used to identify those rootlets that contribute the most to the unbalanced excitatory input on spinal motor neurons. In this way, a usually small portion of the afferent (sensory) fibers can be left intact, thus preserving some sensory function.

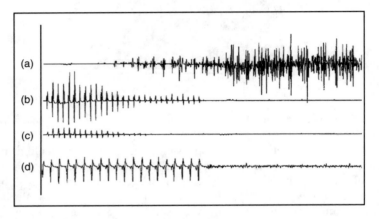

Figure 8.17 Example of EMG activity elicited by a train of 20 stimuli shown in (d). The responses in (a) are abnormal because of after discharges; while those in (b) and (c) are normal because of activity inhibition.

The recording setup involves monitoring triggered EMG from the rectus femoris, tibialis anterior, biceps femoris, and gastrocnemius muscles bilaterally. This setup would cover levels L_2 to S_1, as it can be seen in Table 6.4. Initially, for each rootlet a threshold for eliciting a response is determined using single electrical pulses of successively higher amplitude. Then, the rootlet is stimulated with a train of pulses (usually 20 pulses delivered at a rate of one per second), and a decision regarding the normality of the rootlet is made based on the pattern of activity observed in all muscles. Figure 8.17 shows a typical example of an activity elicited by a train of 20 stimuli.

The following criteria are used to identify abnormal EMG responses and determine which rootlets should be resected. After stimulation, a response is characterized as abnormal if (1) it does not show signs of inhibition, i.e., a train of electrical pulses results in activity of relatively constant amplitude; (2) EMG discharges continue even after stimulation has ceased; (3) there is spread of activity to muscles innervated by adjacent rootlets; and (4) there is crossing of activity to the contralateral side of the body. Usually the rootlets that meet the least number of the above criteria are preserved. In the example of Figure 8.17(a) the response is abnormal because of the presence after discharges, whereas in (b) and (c) the responses are normal, since the recorded activity shows inhibition, i.e., the amplitude of the response to the last few stimuli is drastically reduced.

8.9   Peripheral Nerve Monitoring

8.9.1   Repair of Brachial Plexus

Surgical exploration in the brachial plexus is often necessary to locate and repair nerve damage. The first step in this procedure is to rule out the possibility of a *preganglionic lesion,* i.e., injury near the entry zone of afferent (sensory) fibers into the cervical spine. Surgical repair can only be attempted if the lesion is located distal to the dorsal root ganglion. Preganglionic and postganglionic lesions are depicted in Figure 8.18(a) and Figure 8.18)(b), respectively.

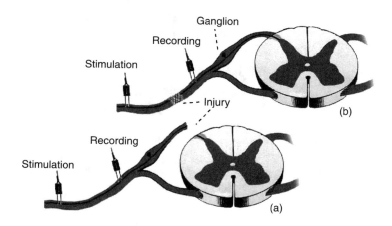

Figure 8.18   (a) Preganglionic and (b) postganglionic lesion in the brachial plexus. Stimulation and recording electrodes used during nerve exploration.

Next, the precise location of the postganglionic lesion must be identified in one of the branches of the brachial plexus or, if it is located more distally, at a peripheral nerve of the arm. Electrophysiological recordings can be particularly helpful in every step of the surgical procedure.

To differentiate a preganglionic from a postganglionic lesion, stimulation of individual nerve roots with a hand-held bipolar stimulator is performed, while recording SEPs from neck and scalp electrodes. The procedure requires minimal averaging, and the resulting SEP latencies are shorter by 7–10 msec compared to the typical responses elicited by stimulation of the same nerve at the wrist. If stimulation of all roots results in well-defined SEPs, then the possibility of a preganglionic lesion is minimal. At this point, a systematic search for the precise location of the postgan-glionic lesion is undertaken, through stimulation and recording over the distal nerve, as shown in Figure 8.18.

During surgical exploration of the brachial plexus, spontaneous EMG can be recorded simultaneously from arm muscles in order to detect potentially harmful nerve irritation.

8.9.2   Acetabular Fixation

Fractures of the pelvis and acetabulum frequently require surgical intervention which typically consists of open reduction and fixation with metal plates. The neural struc-ture at risk during the procedure is the sciatic nerve which traverses the posterior portion of the acetabulum to enter the sacral plexus. A schematic diagram of this arrangement is shown in Figure 8.19.

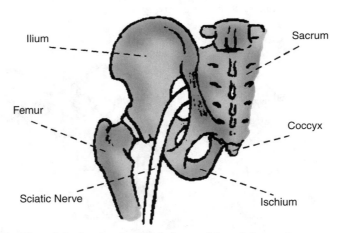

Figure 8.19   The pelvis showing the acetabulum and the sciatic nerve.

The incidence of new or exacerbated nerve injuries associated with this kind of surgery is in the order of 3%, while the most common causes of injury include: (1) compression or abrasion of the nerve by bone fragments, (2) mechanical nerve compression or stretching caused by retraction, changes in the position of the leg during the operation, and insertion of sponges. It should be noted that preexisting damage to the sciatic nerve secondary to the fracture is very common.

The sciatic nerve has two main branches: the posterior tibial and the common peroneal nerves. Thus, its functional integrity can be assessed through posterior tibial SEP recordings. The procedure is described in detail in Section 7.3.4.

Special care should be taken to ensure that the stimulating and recording electrodes in the operated limb, which are placed inside the sterile field, are secure and capable of withstanding the extensive manipulations performed during the operation. Sterile needle EMG electrodes held in place with surgical staples are recommended. If the electrodes are to be placed by the surgeon, then their exact locations should be marked with surgical marker before prepping. After electrode placement the wires and the leg are wrapped in a sterile, self-adhesive elastic bandage.

Monitoring should focus on the cervical and cortical responses, i.e., the responses generated in structures proximal to the site of the surgery. Potential injury to the sciatic nerve can be inferred when stimulation of the operated leg results in a consistent amplitude reduction and possibly a latency prolongation of the cervical and cortical responses while the peripheral response remains unaffected.

Acetabular fixation can be performed using a posterior or anterior approach. The additional risk during the anterior approach is ischemia in the operated leg in the case of an inadvertent occlusion of the femoral artery by a misplaced retractor. The same protocol described above is also used for detecting leg ischemia. In this case, however, the focus of monitoring is on the peripheral response, recorded from the popliteal fossa. Loss of the peripheral response accompanied by loss of the cervical and cortical responses is a reliable index of reduced perfusion of the leg.

8.9.3   Patient Positioning

Improper positioning of the patient on the operating table may carry the risk of nerve damage. For example, prolonged compression of the brachial plexus, when the patient is placed in a prone or lateral position, may result in nerve injury known as *brachial plexopathy*. A schematic diagram of the brachial plexus is shown in Figure 8.20. In most cases, damage to the plexus can be prevented by monitoring the SEPs generated in this region elicited by stimulation of the ulnar nerve, which is more vulnerable than the median.

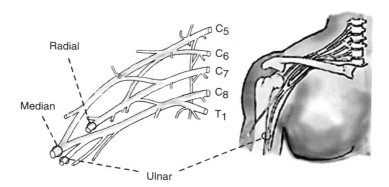

Figure 8.20   Schematic diagram of the brachial plexus showing the location of the vulnerable ulnar nerve.

In addition, improper placement, especially in a prone position, may result in excessive pressure in the abdomen which can compromise the perfusion of the lower extremities and, if prolonged, it may lead to nerve damage. The responses recorded from the popliteal fossa can provide an early warning of vascular damage to the nerves of the lower extremities.

8.10   Review Questions

1. Name the five regions of the spinal cord.

2. What is the spinal canal and what is its function?

3. What is the purpose of stabilization of the spine?

4. Explain what decompression involves.

5. What is spinal fusion?

6. What is the most common approach to spinal surgery?

7. What additional risk does an anterior approach entail?

8. What is the most common test administered for monitoring the spinal cord?

9. What kind of tests can be used to monitor the spine when surgery is above the conus medullaris?

10. What kind of tests can be used to monitor the spine when surgery is below the conus medullaris?

11. What kind of instrumentation is used in the management of scoliosis?

12. During the course of surgery, is the position of a patient on the surgical table important?

13. What does the condition disk herniation entail?

14. What are the typical symptoms of disk herniation?

15. How can ischemia of the cervical spine be differentiated from ischemia of the lumbar spine?

16. What is the major risk in spinal fractures?

17. How are spinal fractures usually corrected?

18. Describe the condition known as spinal stenosis.

19. Which nerve should be stimulated if an operation is above the level of Cvi, at Cvii, or below Cvii cervical vertebra?

20. Describe the condition known as spondylolisthesis.

21. What is the cause of the symptoms usually experienced in a spinal tumor case?

22. What is an aneurysm?

23. What is an AVM?

24. What is the major risk of cross-clamping of the aorta?

25. Which parameter is the most reliable predictor of postoperative deficits in the case of aortic cross-clamping?

26. What does the condition tethered cord entail?

27. What effects does tethered cord have on spinal nerve roots?

28. What is the main purpose of neurophysiological recordings in a tethered cord case?

29. What tests are administered in a tethered cord case?

30. What are the manifestations of spasticity?

31. What does the procedure rhizotomy entail?

32. What tests are administered in a rhizotomy case?

33. In a rhizotomy case, what criteria are used to determine which root should be resected?

34. What is the difference between a preganglionic and a postganglionic lesion in the brachial plexus?

35. What is the most reliable test to determine if an injury is preganglionic?

36. What neural structure is at risk in an acetabular fracture?

37. Why is the setup of tibial nerve SEPs in an acetabular fixation more involved than in other cases?

chapter 9

Cranial Surgery

9.1   Introduction

The human brain can be divided into four main parts, namely the *cerebrum*, the *diencephalon*, the *brainstem*, and the *cerebellum*. In turn, the cerebrum consists of two hemispheres, left and right, each divided into four lobes, *frontal, parietal, temporal,* and *occipital*. The diencephalon is further divided into the thalamus and hypothalamus; whereas, the brainstem consists of three main parts, the mesencephalon, pons, and medulla oblongata. A schematic diagram of the various areas on the surface of the brain is depicted in Figure 9.1.

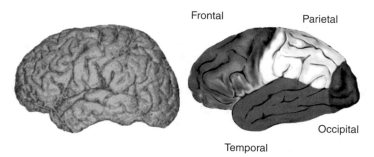

Frontal   Parietal

Occipital

Temporal

Figure 9.1   MRI reconstruction and drawing of the human brain showing the four lobes.

The brain and the spinal cord are covered by three membranes, the *meninges*, that provide protection to the neural tissue. A "folding" in the meninges forms what is known as the *cerebellar tentorium*, which separates the cerebellum from the basal surface of the occipital and temporal lobes. The tentorium is schematically shown in Figure 9.2 enclosed in dashed circles.

Intracranially, the skull forms three incomplete cavities, shown also in Figure 9.2, namely the *anterior fossa* which contains the frontal lobes, the *middle fossa* which contains the temporal and parietal lobes, and the *posterior fossa* which contains the brainstem and the cerebellum. The *cranial base,* the inferior part of the skull, has several foramina (openings) through which cranial nerves and vessels run.

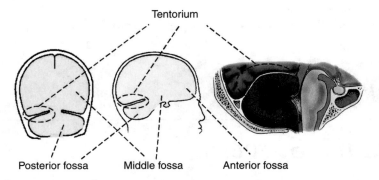

Figure 9.2   Schematic diagram of the anterior, middle, and posterior fossas. The cerebellar tentorium in enclosed by dashed circles.

Most neurosurgical procedures involving the brain are performed to provide relief of symptoms and recovery of impaired neurological function. Some of the most common cases include removal of a tumor (e.g., a schwannoma wrapped around the acoustic nerve), correction of a vascular malformation (e.g., an aneurysm developed in the walls of a major artery), decompression of a cranial nerve (e.g., a blood vessel pressing on the facial nerve), or resection of functionally compromised neural tissue (e.g., removal of an epileptogenic focus in the temporal lobe). In addition, head trauma with local or generalized brain injury often requires immediate surgical intervention.

All of the above surgical procedures include risks that can be classified in two major categories: *mechanical injury* and *ischemia*. Mechanical injury can occur, for instance, during the fine dissection of a tumor from a cranial nerve. Injury can be either direct (i.e., inadvertent trauma) or indirect (e.g., excessive heat generated by the electrocautery unit). On the other hand, ischemia, i.e., a significant reduction of blood supply in a particular brain region, can be caused from prolonged retraction which, in most procedures, is required in order to gain access to the surgical target (e.g., a tumor). Retraction can cause some of the underlying arteries to collapse (especially when the retraction pressure exceeds the systolic blood pressure), thereby reducing local blood flow and, thus, inducing local ischemia.

In most cases, however, both types of complications can be avoided through intraoperative neurophysiological monitoring (IOM), which offers a direct measure of the functional integrity of the neural pathways at risk during an operation. Indeed, in the case, for example, of facial nerve decompression, IOM has been associated with an increased likelihood for preservation of function, which was found to be almost double in monitored versus unmonitored cases [24]. Furthermore, since IOM is performed throughout the course of a procedure, in addition to providing early warnings of an imminent injury, and it can also help in assessing the effectiveness of a corrective surgical intervention.

Table 9.1 summarizes the most common procedures of cranial surgery along with the associated risks and the specific neurophysiological tests that may help reduce these risks.

Table 9.1   Common Procedures of Cranial Surgery, the Associated Risks, and the Specific Neurophysiological Tests that May Help Reduce These Risks

Site of Procedure	Risks	Monitoring
Posterior Fossa: Acoustic neuromas, Aneurysms, AVMs, tumors.	Brainstem ischemia due to occlusion of major vessels (e.g., AICA). Thermal or mechanical damage to ipsilateral cranial nerves V, VII, and VIII (if hearing is intact). Resection of functional neural tissue. Damage to cranial nerves III–XII.	BAERs: peak I and V amplitude, I–V latency difference. SEPs: cortical component amplitude, cervical-cortical component delay. EMG: detect irritation of cranial nerves III–XII. tEMG: identify nerve, test its integrity.
Supratentorium: Aneurysms, AVMs, tumors.	Infarction due to intentional or unintentional occlusion of ACA, ACom, MCA, PCA, or basilar artery. Resection of functional tissue. Rapture of major vessel.	EEG: frontal-central or central-occipital. SEPs (leg or arm stimulation): cortical component amplitude, cervical-cortical component delay.
Microvascular Decompression: Nerves V, VII, and VIII. Partial resection of V nerve	Nerve damage. Damage to motor branch.	BAERs. EMG: detect nerve irritation. tEMG: identify nerve, test its integrity.
Neuroradiological procedures, endarterectomy	Ischemia in the ipsilateral hemisphere.	EEG: frontal-central or central-occipital. SEPs: (arm stimulation).

The most widely employed approach to monitoring the functional integrity of the brain consists of recording somatosensory evoked potentials (SEPs) in response to electrical stimulation of the median nerve at the wrist. SEPs are often supplemented by brainstem auditory evoked responses (BAERs), especially when the VIII cranial nerve or the brainstem itself are at risk. Moreover, monitoring of spontaneous electroencephalographic (EEG) activity provides an excellent measure for detecting the possible onset of ischemia, whereas triggered electromyographic (tEMG) recordings allow to assess the integrity of those cranial nerves that have a motor division.

Chapters 6 and 7 present the standard neurophysiological techniques currently employed for effective monitoring during brain surgery, namely, SEPs, BAERs, EEG, EMG, and tEMG, along with technical details and possible interpretation of the results obtained. In this chapter, we give several specific examples of cranial surgery, whereby intraoperative monitoring has been shown to reduce the risk of long-term postoperative complications.

9.2   Surgery for Tumor Removal

A *tumor* is an abnormal benign or malignant mass of tissue that is not inflammatory, arises without obvious cause from cells of preexistent tissue, and possesses no physiologic function. An example of a brain tumor is shown in the MRI of Figure 9.3, where it appears as a white mass marked with a cross. Medical intervention typically involves resection of the tumor. Depending on the particular case, different neural

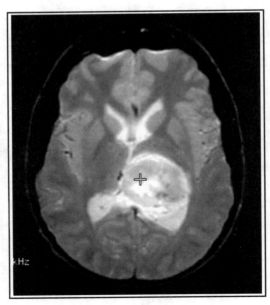

Figure 9.3   Example of a brain tumor marked with a cross.

structures may be at risk. In general, surgical procedures in the brain are categorized according to the anatomical location of the structures involved. The most common locations involved in surgery for tumor are depicted in Figure 9.4.

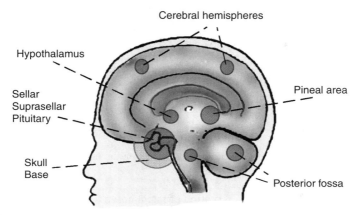

Figure 9.4   Anatomical locations of the most common structures involved in brain surgery.

9.2.1   Posterior Fossa Tumors

One of the most frequent reasons for performing surgery in the posterior fossa is the resection of tumors that wrap around the VIII cranial nerve. These tumors are commonly known as *acoustic neuromas* or *vestibular schwannoma*. Other typical procedures include the removal of tumors that grow on the meninges (i.e., *meningiomas*) and the brainstem itself (i.e., *intrinsic tumors*).

A schematic diagram of the inner ear is depicted in Figure 9.5. The VIII nerve has two branches that follow parallel courses for most of their length: the *auditory* branch which transmits signals from specialized sound receptors in the cochlea, and the *vestibular* branch which carries signals related to the direction of head movement. The latter are generated by the vestibular apparatus. Injury of the auditory branch can result in permanent hearing loss in the ipsilateral and, occasionally, the contralateral ear. On the other hand, injury to the vestibular portion of the nerve can cause dizziness, nystagmus (rhythmic eye movements), nausea, and vomiting.

As an acoustic neuroma expands it may compress or encapsulate a nearby cranial nerve other than the VIII, most commonly the facial (VII) or the trigeminal (V). It may also encapsulate a cerebellar artery, or parts of the brainstem. Thus, additional concerns associated with this procedure include the risk of permanent damage to the VII nerve, which could lead to ipsilateral facial hemiparesis, or the V nerve, which could result in severe ipsilateral facial pain. In addition, vascular intracranial complications, such as hematoma or occlusion of a major vessel, can occur when the vascular supply to the cochlea or the brainstem nuclei is compromised. In severe cases, this may result in brainstem infarction.

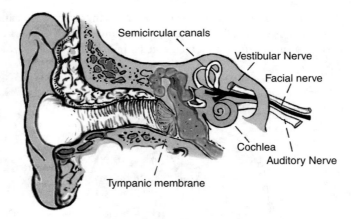

Figure 9.5 Schematic diagram of the inner ear showing the facial, vestibular, and acoustic nerves.

Across studies, the rate of preservation of facial nerve function ranges between 37 and 100%, depending on the size of the tumor and the type of surgical approach followed [15, 25, 50]. In general, nerves may be at greater risk when a translabyrinthine instead of a retrosigmoidal approach is used to expose the acoustic tumor. In that case, the corresponding rates for functional preservation of hearing in the ipsilateral ear are much smaller [25, 50, 63]. The likelihood of hearing preservation is high when the size of the tumor is less than 1.5 cm [33], but the prognosis is not very good with larger tumors.

The entire VIII nerve can be monitored effectively by means of brainstem auditory evoked responses (BAERs) which provide a direct measure of the functional integrity of the auditory pathway. In addition, BAER monitoring offers an indirect measure of the integrity of the vestibular branch, since the two follow the same path before they enter into the brainstem, and they also share a common source of blood supply, namely the interior auditory artery. The exact recording procedure and specific interpretation criteria for BAERs are discussed in Section 7.5.

Depending upon the special characteristics of each case, it may be useful to supplement BAERs with monitoring of the electrophysiological activity of other cranial nerves, especially if a tumor is larger than 2.5 cm in diameter. Procedures for monitoring the facial and trigeminal nerve are described in Section 6.3. Placing needle EMG electrodes in muscles innervated by the motor branches of the nerves under consideration provides recordings that can be used as indices of nerve integrity, since any irritation of a nerve will cause some of the muscle fibers to discharge. Moreover, in cases whereby identification of a nerve is not trivial, direct electrical stimulation of the tissue and observation of the muscle(s) that respond can help in its identification.

A typical application of the last case is the distinction of the facial (VII) from the trigeminal (V) nerve. This information may be crucial in posterior fossa operations, when one of the two nerves is already compromised and the goal is to avoid injury to the intact nerve.

Bipolar electrical stimulation is more specific than monopolar, since there is less current spread, thus this modality is preferable.[1]

When interpreting neurophysiological recordings, EMG activity can be easily confused with various artifacts. To facilitate the task, the EMG signal should be made audible, so that one can listen to its characteristic sound which is reminiscent of "popping popcorn."

An important requirement in all of the procedures that involve EMG monitoring is that the patient is not pharmacologically paralyzed. That is, when checking the level of paralysis, a train of four electrical stimuli, typically delivered to the ulnar or facial nerve, should result in *at least* three muscle contractions.

As previously mentioned, acoustic neuroma cases carry the risk for arterial injury which can lead to brainstem infarction. The artery most closely related to acoustic neuromas is the anterior inferior cerebellar artery (AICA). As Figures 9.7 and 9.12 show, it originates from the basilar artery (BA) and provides blood supply to several structures in the brainstem, including the medial lemniscus, the facial nucleus, and the motor nucleus of the trigeminal nerve. The incidence of brainstem infarctions resulting from injury to the AICA is approximately 2% during translabyrinthine procedures [8].

Occlusion of the AICA or the internal auditory artery can lead to postoperative loss of hearing and facial hemiparesis, even when the VII and VIII nerves have been anatomically preserved. To minimize the risk of ischemia, the above monitoring techniques can be supplemented by median nerve SEPs elicited by stimulation of the hand contralateral to the site of surgery. Details of this procedure are given in Section 7.3.4.

9.2.2 Middle Fossa Tumors

Operations in the middle fossa are performed mostly for the resection of tumors located in the parietal and temporal lobes. In these cases, a sizable proportion of the postoperative neurological complications are caused during surgical exploration, either from damage to functionally intact neural tissue or from cortical ischemia resulting from occlusion of a major vessel. In either case, IOM can play an important role in the prevention of such events.

Standard monitoring procedures should involve recordings of spontaneous EEG and SEPs. For tumors located on the lateral surface of one hemisphere (or in dorsofrontal, parietal, and dorsotemporal areas), median nerve SEPs should be recorded. EEG monitoring should focus on the derivations that lie in close proximity to the exposed cortex. When a tumor is located in the medial surface of one hemisphere, or if it is expected that arteries in the anterior circulation will be at risk during surgical exploration, posterior tibial nerve SEPs should also be monitored. Criteria for

---

[1] If necessary, the functional integrity of the sensory branch of the V nerve can be assessed separately by recording SEPs from the scalp following electrical stimulation of face dermatomes innervated by the trigeminal nerve.

identifying potentially significant changes in the electrophysiological parameters are described in Section 7.3.8.

9.2.3   Anterior Fossa Tumors

Monitoring can also be very useful during surgery for the resection of anterior fossa tumors. These may involve tumors in the frontal lobes, the pituitary gland, etc. Retraction of the frontal lobes to gain access to the tumor is associated with the threat of a vascular insult in the anterior circulation. Monitoring of lower extremity SEPs is the procedure of choice in these cases. However, when retraction involves also the temporal lobe, the addition of upper extremity SEPs is recommended.

For tumors located above the *sella turcica* (suprasellar tumors) concurrent monitoring of both upper and lower extremity SEPs is advisable, because of the proximity of pituitary tumors to the bifurcation of the internal carotid artery, where it divides into the anterior cerebral artery (ACA) and middle cerebral artery (MCA).

During these operations, the optic nerve is also at risk. Thus, recording of visual evoked potential (VEPs) would be necessary. The procedure is described in Section 7.6.4. Unfortunately, in practice intraoperative recordings of VEPs are hindered by a number of technical problems, so that changes in the responses are poorly correlated with the patient's postoperative visual functions. False positives with VEP monitoring are reported to be as high as 95% of the cases [69].

9.2.4   Skull Base Tumors

The primary structures at risk during operations in the area of skull base are the brainstem and the cranial nerves it contains.

Brainstem

The *brainstem* contains neural centers that play a crucial role in the control of sensory, motor, cardiovascular, and respiratory functions. A schematic diagram of this complex structure is given in Figure 9.6.

The brainstem contains nuclei of cranial nerves III to XII and serves as the first relay station for all fibers that carry afferent inputs to the thalamus and the cerebral cortex, such as, for instance, the pyramidal tract. Furthermore, several of its components have fiber connections with the cerebellum. Since all these major neural tracts pass through such a narrow structure, a small lesion in the brainstem may lead to extensive neurologic deficits, and it can even be fatal.

It is possible that surgical manipulations and direct compression of the brainstem may affect the integrity of these structures without causing immediate changes in vital signs, since impaired functions may be temporarily compensated by the various control systems. In that event, neurophysiological parameters are believed to be capable of detecting brainstem insults more rapidly than monitoring of the vital signs alone.

The functional integrity of the auditory and the somatosensory pathways in the brainstem can be monitored directly by means of BAERs and SEPs, respectively. In

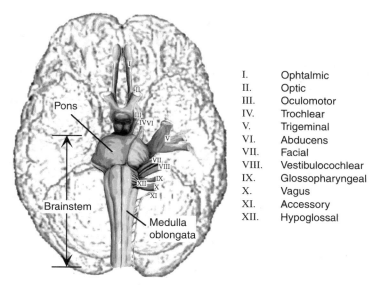

I. Ophtalmic
II. Optic
III. Oculomotor
IV. Trochlear
V. Trigeminal
VI. Abducens
VII. Facial
VIII. Vestibulocochlear
IX. Glossopharyngeal
X. Vagus
XI. Accessory
XII. Hypoglossal

Figure 9.6 Schematic diagram of the brainstem and cranial nerves.

the case of BAERs, due to the extensive crossover of ascending fibers in the upper brainstem, peak V should be recorded following stimulation of each ear separately, provided, of course, that hearing is bilaterally intact. Otherwise, simultaneous bilateral stimulation, or stimulation of only the ear in which hearing is intact, should be performed.

In the case of SEPs, if the structures at risk lie above the level of the medulla (i.e., in the pons or the upper brainstem), then responses to stimulation of the hand *contralateral* to the side of operation are of value. Additionally, in the case of tumors located below the obex of the fourth ventricle, SEPs in response to stimulation of the *ipsilateral* hand should *also* be monitored.

BAER and SEP recordings during a tumor resection have a dual utility. First, they serve as measures of the functional integrity of the neural (auditory and somatosensory) pathways leading to the brainstem which may become compromised due to direct mechanical insult during surgical exploration. Second, these electrophysiological responses can be used as global indices of brainstem integrity and, more specifically, of adequate local blood perfusion. An infarction in this region would most likely affect also structures that either cannot be monitored directly or their monitoring is impractical for routine use. Examples of the latter structure are the sensory nucleus of the trigeminal nerve, the vestibular nuclei, and the abducens nucleus which plays a crucial role in the control of eye movements.

Cranial Nerves

The removal of skull base tumors poses risks for the integrity of cranial nerves that traverse this region (see Figure 9.6). Structures at risk are the III (oculomotor), IV (trochlear), V (trigeminal), VI (abducens), VII (facial), VIII (vestibulocochlear),

IX (glossopharyngeal), X (vagus), XI (spinal accessory), and XII (hypoglossal) nerves, as well as their corresponding brainstem nuclei (e.g., the motor nucleus of the V nerve, the facial nucleus of the VII, etc.). The vestibulocochlear nerve is particularly vulnerable to thermal injury, because it lacks the insulating sheath which forms a protective cover for all the other cranial nerves.

Various neurological deficits are common sequelae of injury to the cranial nerves. In particular, a lesion in the facial nerve can cause total or partial loss of function in the facial muscles and seriously impair eating and speaking. Injury to the motor portion of the trigeminal nerve can lead to severe impairments in mastication. The integrity of the glossopharyngeal nerve is important for certain cardiovascular functions and for swallowing, whereas damage to the vagus nerve can impair vocalization and certain autonomic functions. Injury to the spinal accessory nerve will affect the function of the muscles of the shoulder and neck, whereas injury to the hypoglossal nerve can lead to difficulties in swallowing secondary to atrophy of the tongue muscles. Injury in any of the cranial nerves that innervate the extraocular muscles (oculomotor, trochlear, and abducens nerves) can impair the execution of eye movements. The trochlear and the abducens nerves innervate a single muscle in each eye (the trochlear and the lateral rectus, respectively), whereas the oculomotor nerve innervates four extraocular muscles in each eye. Therefore, injury to the latter can have devastating consequences on the ability to perform eye movements with the affected eye.

All cranial nerves (with the exception of the olfactory, the optic, and the vestibulocochlear) contain motor fibers, while some nerves contain also sensory and autonomic fibers. However, only the motor portion of these nerves is routinely monitored during surgery. Recordings of spontaneous and triggered EMG activity are used to assess the functional integrity not only of the motor division but of an entire nerve. The muscles to use for appropriate monitoring of the various cranial nerves are listed in Table 6.3.

In particular, monitoring of the oculomotor, trochlear, and abducens nerves is a procedure that can be attempted only by specially trained personnel, since extreme care must be taken when placing the needle electrodes in the inferior oblique, superior oblique,[2] and lateral rectus muscles, in order to avoid damaging the eye.

The criteria for identifying spontaneous EMG activity that may have prognostic value for postoperative function of the monitored nerve have been described in Section 6.3.6.

9.3   Neurovascular Procedures

The distribution of blood vessels in the brain is really extensive. The most important of these arteries is schematically shown in Figure 9.7, while Figure 9.8 depicts the two main supplies to the brain, namely the carotid and the vertebral arteries.

---

[2]All motor cranial nerves innervate muscles in the *ipsilateral* side, with the exception of the trochlear nerve, in which some fibers innervate the contralateral superior oblique muscle.

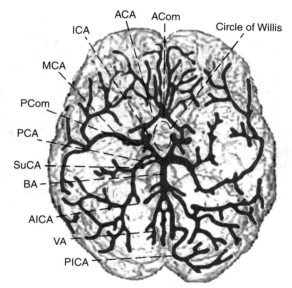

Figure 9.7 Distribution of the most important arteries in the brain.

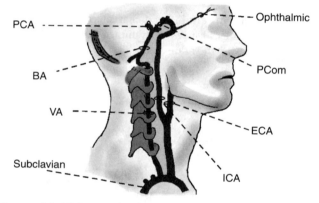

Figure 9.8 The carotid and the vertebral arteries are the main blood supplies to the brain.

Neurovascular procedures entail surgical intervention in blood vessels in the nervous system, and in particular, the brain. Probably the most common procedures are resection of an *arteriovenous malformation* (AVM) and clipping of an *aneurysm*. As mentioned in Section 8.6, AVMs are abnormal communications between arteries and veins whereby blood is shunted directly from the arterial system to the venous system. Figures 9.9(a) and Figure 9.9(b) show two examples of AVM involving areas supplied by the internal carotid artery (ICA) and by vessels of the posterior circulation, respectively.

An aneurysm, on the other hand, is an abnormal dilation of an artery that presents the potential risk of rupture and clotting. Intracranial aneurysms are usually *saccular*

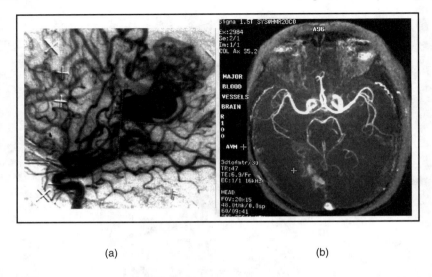

(a)   (b)

Figure 9.9 Examples of arteriovenous malformations involving (a) areas supplied by the internal carotid and (b) the posterior circulation.

(have the form of a mushroom) exhibiting a characteristic neck, as is schematically shown in Figure 9.10. Figure 9.11 gives an example of a large aneurysm in the basilar artery that is also compressing the brainstem.

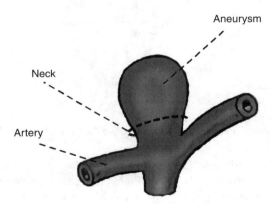

Figure 9.10 A schematic diagram of a saccular aneurysm and its characteristic neck.

The threat of ischemia in functionally intact brain tissue is especially high during these procedures, because they often involve intentional, temporary or permanent, clipping of several feeding vessels. That is, before the application of the permanent clip, the surgeon will typically test the importance of a vessel by first applying a temporary clip that is relatively easy to remove.

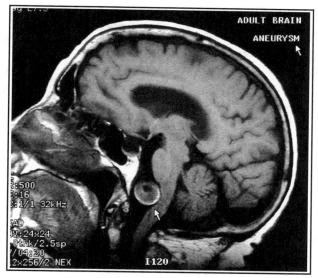

Figure 9.11 Example of a large aneurysm (arrow) involving the basilar artery.

Thus, in general, vascular operations carry the risk of brain ischemia which can be caused by several reasons including: (1) brain retraction, used to achieve adequate exposure of the aneurysm; (2) partial or complete occlusion of an artery by a misplaced clip, this is most likely to occur in large aneurysms with a short neck; and (3) unintentional perforation of a vessel that lies near the aneurysm by a temporary or permanent clip. The structures at risk and the most appropriate tests to administer depend on the surgical site.

9.3.1 Posterior Fossa Aneurysms

The most common sites of aneurysms in the posterior fossa are the posterior inferior cerebellar artery (PICA), the anterior inferior cerebellar artery (AICA), the superior cerebellar artery (SuCA), the basilar (BA), and the vertebral arteries, which are depicted in Figure 9.7 and in more detail in Figure 9.12. Standard monitoring procedures involve the simultaneous recording of BAERs and median nerve SEPs. Auditory stimulation should be performed ipsilateral *and* contralateral to the side of the operation. Monitoring should focus on the amplitude of peaks I and V, and the I–V interpeak latency. In the case of aneurysms in the SuCA and AICA, somatosensory stimulation should be delivered to the hand *contralateral* to the side of the operation. Conversely, during monitoring of PICA aneurysms, SEPs elicited by stimulation of the *ipsilateral* hand are of primary importance.

As it has been explained earlier, the SEP parameters that have the highest prognostic value are the amplitude and latency of the cortical component (N20–P25) and the central conduction time (CCT). A sudden deterioration in these parameters is generally more significant than a gradual change. The surgical team should be warned

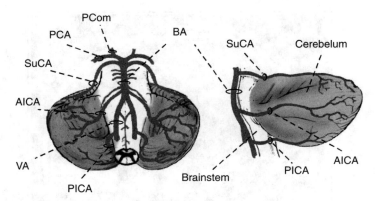

Figure 9.12   Distribution of the basilar artery (BA) in the posterior fossa.

immediately if degradation of the responses occurs within a few minutes after placement of a retractor, or a permanent or temporary clip, so that they can take immediate
action. Repositioning the retractor or the clip is usually sufficient to ensure recovery
of the electrophysiological responses.

Another potential complication during posterior fossa surgery is the occurrence of
air emboli, especially when a sitting position is used. The incidence of air emboli in
the sitting position may be as high as 25% [64] or even 30% [76] of all the cases, and
it can have serious neurological sequelae if undetected.

9.3.2   Brainstem and Skull Base

The resection of tumors and AVMs located in the brainstem and skull base is associated with potentially serious surgical complications. Major factors that contribute
to postoperative morbidity include resection of functionally intact neural tissue and
mechanical or vascular insult to brainstem nuclei and pathways. Operations in the
cerebellopontine angle may compromise the blood supply to the brainstem by reducing the blood flow through the vertebral, BA, PICA, AICA, SuCA, or the posterior
cerebral artery (PCA). Large tumors or meningiomas may compress, displace, or
encase one or more of these large vessels. During tumor removal, major arteries
may become occluded (by retraction) or injured, leading to ischemia in brain regions
supplied by these vessels.

9.3.3   Supratentorial Procedures

Posterior Circulation

In this section we describe monitoring procedures for aneurysms located in the internal
carotid artery (ICA), the middle cerebral artery (MCA), the posterior cerebral artery
(PCA), the posterior communicating artery (PCom), and the rostral part of the basilar
(BA) artery, including the basilar tip. These vessels are schematically shown in
Figure 9.7 and in more detail in Figures 9.13 and 9.14.   In these cases, standard
monitoring procedures involve continuous recordings of EEG and median nerve SEPs.

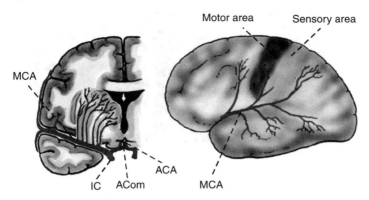

Figure 9.13   Distribution of the middle cerebral artery (MCA) in the brain.

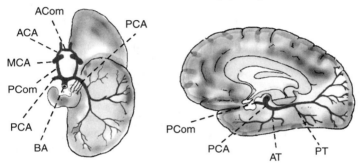

Figure 9.14   Distribution of the posterior communicating artery (PCA) in the brain.

Criteria for identifying potentially significant changes in the parameters of ongoing EEG can be found in Section 6.2.8. The hand area of the primary somatosensory cortex falls in the distribution of ICA and MCA. Therefore, occlusion of one of these arteries is expected to cause dramatic changes in the cortical component of the median nerve SEP. Normally, however, the reduction of blood flow is compensated by collateral blood supply or by blood flow from the contralateral ICA, through the *circle of Willis,* a structure formed by several arteries across the two hemispheres, as shown in Figures 9.7 and 9.15.

Occlusion of the PCA may also cause SEP changes due to reduced perfusion in the region of the medial lemniscus, which is supplied by short peripheral branches of PCA, and thalamus, primarily supplied by the thalamogeniculate branches of PCA. In these cases, monitoring should focus on components recorded from the site *ipsilateral* to the side of surgery (i.e., C_3' in a left craniotomy and C_4' in a right craniotomy) in response to stimulation of the *contralateral* hand.

Comparison of SEP parameters between sides is particularly useful as a means for ascertaining that an occasional change is due to iatrogenic (surgical manipulation) rather than perisurgical factors, such as, for example, a bolus injection of an anesthetic agent. The effects of the former are expected to be restricted to the side ipsilateral to surgery, while changes associated with perisurgical factors are most likely to occur

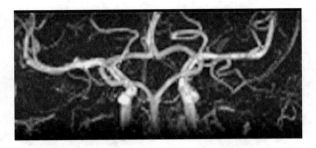

Figure 9.15   Several interconnected arteries across the two hemispheres form the circle of Willis.

bilaterally. An exception to this rule concerns midline aneurysms, such as aneurysms located on the basilar artery. Occlusion of this vessel is likely to cause ischemia in both hemispheres. Given that the basilar artery is the primary source of the posterior circulation, significant disruption of blood flow through this artery is expected to cause drastic SEP changes.

Anterior Circulation

The procedures described in this section involve the clipping of aneurysms located in the anterior cerebral artery (ACA) or the anterior communicating artery (ACom). A schematic diagram of the distribution of these arteries shown in Figure 9.16. Clipping

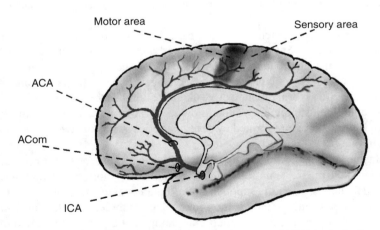

Figure 9.16   Distribution of the anterior communicating artery (ACA) in the brain.

of an aneurysm in the ACom may affect the blood flow in both ACAs. However, one should be aware that the function of structures supplied by small branches of ACA and ACom, such as the ophthalmic and the hypothalamic branches, cannot be effectively monitored using the currently available techniques.

The ACA is the main source of blood supply to the leg area of the primary somatosensory cortex. The cortical SEP elicited by stimulation of the contralateral posterior tibial nerve is used as an index of brain perfusion in the distribution of the ACA (specifically, of the callosomarginal and pericallosal branches of the ACA). Typically, a combination of SEPs and EEG is employed. EEG monitoring is especially important if the aneurysm is located in the frontopolar branches of the ACA.

Procedures involving these areas may also entail retraction of the temporal lobe, a manipulation that may lead to partial obstruction of blood flow through the MCA and one or more of its branches. This artery is the main source of blood supply to (the hand area of) the somatosensory cortex, the functional integrity of which can be monitored via SEPs elicited by stimulation of the median nerve. Thus, during vascular procedures in the anterior circulation, monitoring should include the cortical responses elicited by stimulation of both the lower and the upper extremities.

If the available monitoring equipment does not permit simultaneously recording of upper and lower extremity SEPs, an alternative monitoring strategy can be used. Initially, a few traces of SEPs elicited by posterior tibial and median nerve stimulation should be recorded for use as baselines. During the surgical exploration that aims at exposing the aneurysm, median nerve SEPs should be used to ensure that perfusion of the brain following retraction of the temporal lobe is not seriously compromised. EEG monitoring should focus on recordings from centro-occipital derivations. When the surgeon has achieved adequate exposure, monitoring should be switched to lower extremity SEPs, and EEG monitoring should concentrate primarily on recordings from frontocentral derivations.

EEG events should be considered significant if they are focal, i.e., localized in centro-occipital derivations in the case of posterior circulation aneurysms, and in frontocentral derivations in the case of anterior circulation aneurysms.

9.4 Cranial Nerve Surgery

Surgery targeted to cranial nerves is used for the management of a number of conditions associated with impaired nerve function, which can be vascular or nonvascular in origin. *Microvascular decompression* is one such procedure used for the management of acute localized pain and involuntary muscle spasm, which is often caused by the compression of a cranial nerve by blood vessels as it enters the brainstem. In this procedure, the vessel responsible for nerve compression is separated from the nerve by inserting a small piece of soft insulating material. Cranial nerves commonly suffering from this condition are the trigeminal (V), facial (VII), vestibulocochlear (VIII), and glossopharyngeal (IX).

The vessels most frequently responsible for trigeminal nerve compression, which results in acute intractable facial pain known as *trigeminal neuralgia,* are the anterior cerebral artery (ACA) and, less frequently, the anterior inferior cerebellar artery (AICA). Conversely, the posterior inferior cerebellar artery (PICA) and, less frequently, AICA have been implicated in cases of vascular compression of the facial nerve causing hemifacial spasm. Vascular compression of the VIII nerve is often responsible for hearing impairment, tinnitus (persistent ringing of the ear), impaired equilibrium, and vertigo. Finally, glossopharyngeal neuralgia is a far less common condition than trigeminal neuralgia and hemifacial spasm, and its causes are largely unknown. Treatment may involve partial resection of the nerve.

Another condition associated with impaired cranial nerve function is facial paralysis. This impairment is of nonvascular origin and its surgical treatment involves identification and repair of the damaged portion of the facial nerve.

Intraoperative monitoring of spontaneous and triggered EMG (tEMG) from the orbicularis oris and frontalis muscles is recommended during microvascular decompression procedures performed to relieve hemifacial spasm. Details on this procedure can be found in Section 6.3.6.

Besides allowing the identification of a nerve, recordings of tEMG can have an additional utility in this operation. Direct electrical stimulation of the temporal branch of the facial nerve elicits an abnormal response that shows a characteristically prolonged latency (approximately 10 msec) and is followed by afterdischarges. This response is preferably obtained from the frontalis muscle after the patient is anesthetized [49]. A dramatic reduction in the amplitude of the abnormal response is usually observed after the facial nerve is separated from the vessel responsible for the compression. If the characteristics of the response remain unchanged, then there is a good chance that a second vessel is also compressing the nerve.

During operations targeted to cranial nerves V and VII, the VIII nerve is also at risk, due to the proximity of these structures (see Figure 9.5). Postoperative preservation of hearing in the ipsilateral ear is a major concern in these procedures. Thus, in these cases, ipsilateral BAER monitoring is advisable.

Another type of procedure involves resection of the sensory branch of the trigeminal nerve in order to control severe cluster headaches. Monitoring of both spontaneous and triggered EMG is strongly recommended also in these procedures. The responses to direct nerve stimulation (tEMG) can be used for differentiating the trigeminal from the facial nerve, since stimulation of the trigeminal nerve elicits a response in the masseter, but not in the orbicularis oris, orbicularis oculi, or frontalis muscles.

Also, tEMG can be used to identify and thus avoid damage to the motor branch of the nerve which must be preserved. In addition to tEMG, continuous recording of spontaneous EMG can be used to provide early warnings of mechanical or thermal irritation of the nerve. Finally, periodic stimulation of the trigeminal nerve and recording of tEMG can inform the surgeon of the functional integrity of the nerve at any given point in time.

Successive tracings of tEMG signals should allow the detection of changes in the amplitude of the response over time. Since the response amplitude reflects the number of nerve fibers that are recruited by the electrical stimulus, an amplitude reduction suggests that nerve conduction is partially blocked at a certain part of the nerve. A prolonged reduction in response amplitude that is not due to perisurgical events, such as an increased level of muscle relaxation, is associated with an increased likelihood of postoperative muscle weakness.

9.5 Endarterectomy

The internal carotid artery (ICA), one on each side, arises from the common carotid artery and serves as a major source of blood supply to the brain. The ICA gives rise to the middle cerebral (MCA) and the anterior cerebral arteries (ACA). Carotid endarterectomy is often required in order to remove atheromatous plaques that adhere on the lining of the ICA.

In many cases this surgical procedure is deemed necessary for the prevention of neurological symptoms, such as transient ischemic attacks and stroke caused by reduced blood flow to the brain. The procedure requires cross-clamping of the artery, dissection of the vessel and removal of the plaque, and closure of the incision. A schematic diagram of this procedure is shown in Figure 9.17.

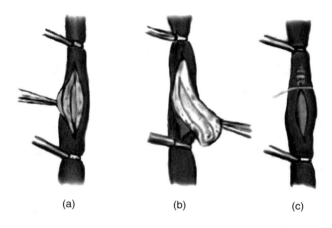

(a)   (b)   (c)

Figure 9.17 Schematic diagram of a carotid endarterectomy procedure. (a) Cross-clamping and dissection of the internal carotid, (b) removal of plaque, and (c) closure of the incision.

In most cases, adequate blood flow to brain regions normally supplied by the clamped vessel is maintained from contralateral vessels through the circle of Willis (see Figure 9.7). Occasionally, however, contralateral circulation is not sufficient to compensate for the disrupted blood flow, and cross-clamping of ICA will cause ischemia in several brain regions. An example of this is shown in Figure 9.18. Short after arterial clamping (time 9:41), a significant reduction in the peak-to-peak amplitude of the SEP component was observed (time 9:45) which was further decreasing (time 9:55), indicating severe ischemia. Placement of a shunt, however, restores adequate blood supply and the response returns to normal (time 10:01).

A standard monitoring protocol that has proven to be effective in providing early warnings of ischemia involves continuous monitoring of EEG (from at least three bipolar derivations on each side), and median nerve SEPs. Ischemia induced by occlusion of the ICA is expected to cause a sudden reduction in the amplitude of the high frequency EEG rhythms. EEG changes should be restricted to the frontocentral

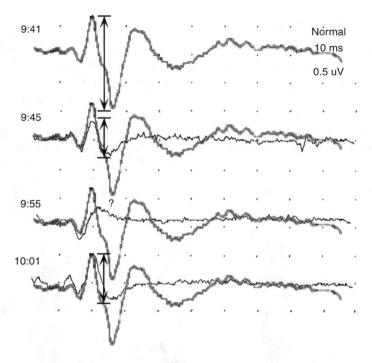

Figure 9.18 SEPs obtained after cross-clamping of the internal carotid (time 9:41) which resulted in ischemia (time 9:45) that later deteriorated (9:55). After placement of a shunt, response amplitude is restored to within normal limits (time 10:01).

derivation in the hemisphere ipsilateral to the operated side. SEP monitoring should focus on central conduction time (CCT) and the amplitude of the cortical component, which is presumably generated in the somatosensory strip, a region supplied by MCA.

9.6   Neuroradiological Procedures

Interventional radiological techniques have several diagnostic and therapeutic applications. Procedures that are most commonly performed with neurophysiological monitoring are those involving embolization of AVMs and occlusion, either temporary or permanent, of a vessel. Vessel occlusion is achieved using an inflatable balloon that is inserted into a large artery (typically the femoral artery of the leg) with the aid of a catheter and continuous X-ray imaging. A schematic diagram of this procedure is shown in Figure 9.19.

Occlusion procedures may be diagnostic (for instance, to determine if a given vessel can be sacrificed in an upcoming operation without causing cerebral infarction), or therapeutic (for instance, performed in order to cutoff the blood supply to an AVM). However, embolization procedures are commonly used to reduce the size of AVMs preoperatively, and facilitate their surgical resection. The primary risk associated

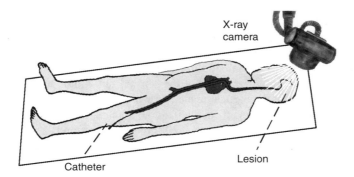

Figure 9.19   Embolization of an AVM using a balloon inserted into the femoral artery of the leg under continuous X-ray imaging.

with both procedures is a significant reduction in blood flow in the distal part of the artery leading to damage of healthy neural tissue from ischemia.

Electrophysiological monitoring is used to ensure that the brain regions normally supplied by the occluded vessel are adequately perfused by collateral circulation throughout the procedure. Available monitoring procedures include SEPs, BAERs, and EEG. A combination of EEG and SEPs is used if the interventional target is a supratentorial vessel. Median nerve SEPs should be monitored if arteries involved are the ICA, MCA, PCA, PCom, or BA. Posterior tibial nerve SEPs should be used when the procedure involves the ACA or the ACom artery. Conversely, a combination of SEPs and BAERs is the method of choice in procedures that involve brainstem vessels.[3] Interpretation criteria are similar to those described in previous sections in the context of monitoring procedures for aneurysm clipping.

9.7   *Central Sulcus Localization*

In several cases, the precise localization of the *central sulcus,* the borderline between the motor (precentral) and somatosensory (postcentral) cortical areas, is essential. For instance, individuals suffering from medically intractable epilepsy may have to undergo surgical treatment to remove the affected brain tissue. If the epileptogenic focus is in the somatosensory cortex near the central sulcus, resection of tissue in the precentral gyrus may result in unwanted motor deficits. On the other hand, concerns about such deficits may lead to inadequate surgical intervention. Similar concerns can be expressed for tumor patients when the lesion is located, for example, in the frontoparietal junction.

Therefore, precise identification of the sulcus is crucial in order to avoid the resection of functionally intact tissue which could lead to severe postoperative deficits.

---

[3]Occasionally, the target is one of the spinal arteries, in which case, SEPs should be used (median nerve stimulation for C_1–C_6 levels, ulnar nerve stimulation for C_6–C_7 levels, and posterior tibial nerve stimulation for levels lower than C_7).

Because of the large intrasubject variability in regional anatomy, visual identification alone of the central sulcus may lead to erroneous conclusions.

Intraoperative procedures for localizing the somatosensory cortex include the recording of median nerve SEPs obtained directly from the exposed cortex. SEPs can be used to delineate precisely the extent of the sensory and motor areas, because of a characteristic feature of the cortical responses which show phase reversal across the central sulcus, i.e., the latency of individual components is preserved whereas their polarity is reversed, as shown in Figure 9.20. Polarity inversion is a well-established and highly-reliable criterion for the identification of the central sulcus.

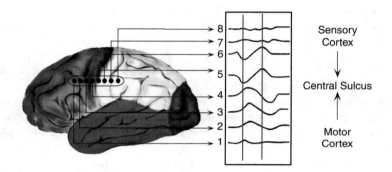

Figure 9.20   Central sulcus identification through median nerve SEPs recorded on the surface of the exposed cortex. Note the component reversal between electrodes 4 and 5.

9.8   Review Questions

1. Name the four lobes in which each brain hemisphere can be divided.

2. What is the name of the membrane covering the brain and the spinal cord?

3. What is the cerebellar tentorium?

4. Give the names of the three cavities formed in the skull.

5. What kind of risks does brain retraction entail?

6. What is the most common neurophysiological recording performed in brain surgery?

7. What is a tumor?

8. What cranial nerves are at risk in an acoustic neuroma procedure?

9. What tests are administered in an acoustic neuroma procedure?

10. Which artery is most closely related to acoustic neuromas?

11. What are the potential risks from injury of the AICA?

12. Which brain structures does the middle fossa contain?

13. What tests are administered in a middle fossa case?

14. Which brain structures does the anterior fossa contain?

15. What tests are administered in an anterior fossa case?

16. What brain structures are at risk during operations in the skull base?

17. What is the primary test administered to monitor the brainstem?

18. When monitoring the brainstem through BAERs, which peak is the most important?

19. What are the primary symptoms of an injury to the seventh cranial nerve?

20. What are the primary symptoms of an injury to the fifth cranial nerve?

21. What is the primary test to monitoring cranial nerves?

22. What are the most common neurovascular procedures?

23. What kind of tests are administered in posterior fossa cases?

24. What are the most important vessels involved in supratentorial procedures?

25. Give the name of the vessel structure that allows circulation of the blood from one hemisphere to the other.

26. What is the most appropriate test to administer during a PCA aneurysm?

27. What is the most appropriate test to administer during a AICA aneurysm?

28. What is the most appropriate test to administer during a PICA aneurysm?

29. What is the most appropriate test to administer during a BA aneurysm?

30. What is the most appropriate test to administer during a ACom aneurysm?

31. What is the most appropriate test to administer during a ACA aneurysm?

32. What is the most appropriate test to administer during cranial nerve surgery?

33. Describe the carotid endarterectomy procedure.

34. What test is recommended for monitoring a carotid endarterectomy procedure?

35. What is the purpose of an embolization procedure?

36. What tests are recommended for supratentorial procedures in posterior circulation vessels?

37. What tests are recommended for supratentorial procedures in anterior circulation vessels?

38. Describe the central sulcus localization procedure.

chapter 10

Artifacts and Troubleshooting

10.1   Introduction

The purpose of intraoperative monitoring is to detect the onset of changes in the functional status of neurological structures that could result in permanent postoperative neurological deficits, so that actions can be taken early enough to reverse the offense and restore normal function. The efficacy of intraoperative monitoring (IOM) depends on the *sensitivity* and *specificity* of the criteria used for interpretation of the recordings, i.e., on their ability to detect true changes *accurately* and differentiate them from false alarms. Exact interpretation criteria for each test administered can be found in Chapters 6 and 7.

During the monitoring procedure, artifactual changes can happen because of electrical noise, changes in anesthesia regime, interference from extraneous neurophysiological activity such as the ECG, and equipment failure. Because of all these factors, and the fact that neurophysiological signals normally vary over time, successful IOM depends on the ability to differentiate changes that are due to surgical intervention, the so-called *iatrogenic* factors, from changes that are independent of surgical maneuvers, and they are known as *perisurgical* factors.

10.2   Efficacy of Monitoring

The objective of proper IOM is to maximize the overall *success rate* (i.e., to detect and report real changes and identify and disregard artifacts). This can be achieved by minimizing the *false negatives* (i.e., real changes that have been erroneously classified as nonsignificant) and the *false positives* (i.e., normal changes that have been erroneously classified as significant). This approach will result in fewer postoperative complications and fewer unnecessary warnings to the surgeon who, after several false alerts, may lose confidence in the validity of, or the necessity for, the IOM service. Thus, the personnel involved in administering the various IOM tests should be familiar and able to deal with the different kinds of artifacts that are often encountered in the operating room.

10.3   *Artifacts*

In general, the operating room is a "hostile" environment for recording electrophysiological activity because of the large number of different machines used and the high level of electrical noise they produce. Besides the ubiquitous 60 Hz electrical interference caused by the power lines, all pieces of equipment generate various types of noise whose effects range from simple "smearing" in some neurophysiological signals, to complete obliteration of all recordings.

For instance, the *bovie* (an electrocautery device used for cutting and coagulation) and the *CUSA* (which is used to debulge tumors by pulsating water at ultrasonic frequencies) are the most notorious devices as they completely prevent monitoring during their use. Other devices, such as the *cell saver* (which recycles the patient's blood lost during surgery), the *bare hugger* (used to keep the patient warm by circulating hot air in an inflated plastic blanket placed over the patient), the blood warmer, the microscope, the surgeon's head lights, and the operating table, all will introduce more or less noise, depending on their proximity to the recording electrodes and the (pre)amplifiers. Other artifacts can result from extraneous neurophysiological signals (such as muscle and cardiac activity), from changes in anesthesia regime (due to, for instance, a bolus injection of an anesthetic agent), and from changes in blood pressure or body temperature. Since the electrophysiologist or technologist administering the tests has usually little control over these artifacts, it is necessary to minimize their effects on the test results.

An example of different kinds of artifacts is shown in Figure 10.1. The four spikes in trace (a) are due to the stimulation of the facial nerve by the anesthesiologist to determine the patient's level of muscle relaxation, as described in Section 5.7.1. The artifacts in trace (b) and (c) are generated by the surgical table and the surgeon's headlight, respectively, while the high frequency noise of trace (d) is due to the bipolar electrocautery device. Notice that in all cases the neurophysiological signals have completely disappeared.

10.4   *Precautions*

One should plan ahead and take all possible precautions to avoid at least some simple technical problems, such as disconnected electrodes and excessive electrical interference.

To this end, during the setup, the recording electrodes (typically subdermal needles) should be secured on the patient's head with tape (or even with surgical staples when movement of the head is expected), to avoid changes in electrode impedance and electrode detachment. To minimize electrical interference, electrodes should be as short as possible and away from tubes, wires, neurostimulators, or any other anesthesia piece of equipment which typically lies close to the patient's head. Sometimes, it helps to braid electrodes together so that all follow the same pathway to the headbox and, therefore, they are all affected by the same type and amount of noise. In that case, the differential amplifiers, under the ideal conditions mentioned in Section 3.7.5, would reject the common interference signal, thus allowing only biological activity to be

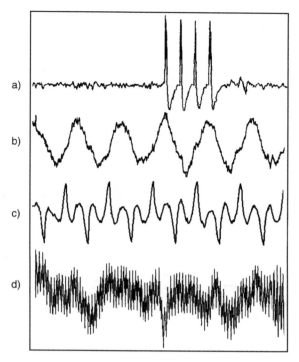

Figure 10.1   Examples of artifacts generated by (a) a neurostimulator, (b) the surgical table, (c) the surgeon's head light, and (d) the bipolar electrocautery device.

recorded. Moreover, whenever possible, all parts of the monitoring equipment, such as amplifiers and nerve stimulators, should be positioned in such a way so that they remain readily accessible after draping of the patient, should the need for accessing the equipment arises.

It is also important that the neurophysiologist responsible for monitoring discuss the test administered with the anesthesiologist and ask for a regime as steady as possible. From the monitoring point of view, administration of drugs in drip infusion (instead of bolus injections), and blood pressure control with vasoactive agents (rather than by changing the level of inhalational anesthetic, such as Isoflurane), are preferred, because they provide a much more stable regime throughout the operation. Also, depending on the case, maintaining a constant muscle relaxation level, possibly through a drip infusion, is highly desirable.

Another precaution that can help tremendously during troubleshooting is the recording strategy itself, which should include multiple recording sites. For instance, the recommended montage for somatosensory evoked potentials includes one cortical, one cervical, and one peripheral response for each side of the body. If a change is detected, examination of the pathway between the stimulation site, the distal response (before the incision), and the proximal response (after the incision), can provide information as to the origin of the change.

Being aware of the patients clinical status helps as well. For instance, in patients with peripheral neuropathies, the nerves should be stimulated more proximally to reduce the distance that the electrical stimulus has to travel and, thus, the total resistance it has to overcome. Thus, in this example, to monitor posterior tibial nerve responses, one should use the popliteal fossa as a stimulation site instead of the ankle. This would result in more robust and more reliable responses.

10.5   Troubleshooting

Once a change that meets criteria for significance has been detected[1] it is necessary to follow a methodical strategy in order to determine the cause of the change. First, it must be established whether the change is real or artifactual and, then, whether it is due to perisurgical or iatrogenic factors. An organized approach to troubleshooting can be summarized in the following steps:

1. Determine the reliability of the change. For nonaveraged signals, a change is reliable if it is persistent over time, whereas for averaged responses, a change is reliable if it can be replicated at least twice in a row and both repetitions differ significantly from baseline.

2. Identify the origin of the change by establishing whether the peripheral, cervical, cortical, or all three responses are degraded or missing.

3. Check for technical problems, such as an increase in electrode impedance, electrical interference, or faulty (electrical or auditory) stimulators.

4. Check for perioperative causes, such as muscle artifacts, drug administration, or a decrease in body temperature or blood pressure.

5. Correlate the observed changes with surgical maneuvers.

6. If none of the previous attempts can explain the degraded responses, the change can be considered real. At this point both the surgeon and the anesthesiologist should be informed of the observed changes.

When troubleshooting for technical causes (Step 3 in the previous list) one should check that:

1. All electrodes are placed securely on the patient and show a low impedance, and that the amplifiers are turned on and functioning correctly.

2. Adequate stimulation is being delivered to the patient. For example, in the case of SEPs, one should check the amplitude of the peripheral responses recorded at the popliteal fossa or the Erb's point. Sometimes, excessive patient perspiration

---

[1]As mentioned before, in the case, for example, of SEPs a 50% change in the amplitude and/or a 10% change in the latency constitutes a significant change.

causes poor contact between the stimulating electrodes and the skin. It is also possible that one of the stimulating devices malfunctions and it cannot deliver a full strength stimulus. In this case, switching the connections between the left and right side electrodes should cause the change to appear in the responses of the opposite side.

Similarly, in the case of ABRs, a stable peak I indicates appropriate stimulus delivery. If the ear canal gets blocked by fluids from the surgical field, the responses may degrade or even disappear. To check for a possible hardware failure, again the left and right side stimulators could be switched.

3. No new equipment that could generate electrical interference has been placed near the recording electrodes or amplifiers.

If the cause of response degradation can be attributed to the presence of excessive noise, the nature of the interference can be determined by inspecting the input signal, i.e., the single-trial responses. If the interference is periodic, as in the case of 60 Hz cycle from power lines, it is possible to change the stimulation rate so that averaging is not synchronized to the external noise. A small change in the stimulation rate, for example from the typical value of 4.7 Hz to 4.6 Hz, should cause the noise signal to appear with a different phase in individual trials (the noise signal should appear to "march" across the screen as individual trials are collected) and, thus, it should cancel out with averaging.

If the interference is not periodic, using a slower stimulation rate, for example 2.1 Hz instead of the typical 4.7 Hz, or increasing the stimulus intensity, say from 25 mA to 35 mA, would result in a stronger response in every single trial and, thus, the signal-to-noise ratio in the average response would be increased.

10.6   Intervention

When a change has been identified as real (by excluding all other possibilities) and the surgeon and anesthesiologist have been notified, depending on the nature of the operation, the time in the course of the procedure, and the specific change observed, the surgeon may decide to ignore the warning, if there is no apparent reason for the change to have happened. On the other hand, if the change in the neurophysiological signals correlates with a surgical maneuver, the surgeon may elect to take one or several of the following corrective actions: (1) release retracted tissues; (2) remove surgical clips and release occluded vessels; (3) remove corrective farces that provide distraction and derotation; (4) remove hardware instrumentation, including hooks, screws, rods, and plates.

Typically, the above actions reverse the offending action and the degraded neurophysiological signals return to baseline values. However, if the signals do not improve, or if they continue to degrade, the surgeon may choose to administer the so-called *wake-up test* (see next section) to examine directly the functional integrity of the nervous system.

It is very important that neurophysiological monitoring be continued, if possible, during *all* corrective actions, so that the effects of each action can be evaluated. If the above intervention restores the signals, and this is confirmed by a wake-up test, this will increase the surgeon's confidence in monitoring.

Another common intraoperative intervention is the administration of steroids, although their neuroprotective efficacy in intraoperative ischemia has not been established unequivocally.

10.7   The Wake-up Test

The ultimate intraoperative test of nervous system function is the "wake-up test," which evaluates the functional integrity of neuronal structures directly (as opposed to the indirect evaluation provided by neurophysiological monitoring). The wake-up test can assure the integrity of neuronal structures, at least at the time it is administered. During the test, anesthetic agents are temporarily discontinued, muscle paralysis is reversed, and blood pressure, which usually is decreased during surgery to reduce bleeding, is brought back to normal values. Only administration of oxygen is continued. The patient emerges from anesthesia enough to follow commands, such as toe or foot movement, and hand squeeze. If these movements can be performed, the test is considered negative for paraplegia, and the patient is reanesthetized to complete the surgery.

Another advantage of the wake-up procedure is that, if the changes that lead to the administration of the test resulted from ischemia, the increased blood pressure may provide the necessary tissue perfusion to restore neuronal function. However, there are two major disadvantages associated with this test: (1) it only provides *momentary* information about the integrity of the nervous system, and (2) this information regards only *voluntary* movements. Because of these problems, along with the fact that patient's amnesia to this unpleasant experience cannot be guaranteed, and the additional effort and time needed, the wake-up test is less commonly practiced today than it has been in the past, however, some centers still consider it as the "gold standard." Instead, it is administered only if electrophysiological monitoring is not available or when the results provided are confusing.

10.8   Review Questions

1. What kinds of artifacts affect the IOM recordings?

2. How can the success rate of IOM be improved?

3. What two pieces of equipment create such an interference that renders IOM impossible?

4. What kind of precautions should be taken during setup to minimize electrical interference?

5. What strategy should be followed to determine the cause of an observed change?

6. State the steps to follow when troubleshooting for technical reasons.

7. Describe briefly the wake-up test.

8. When is the wake-up test administered?

chapter 11

Closing Remarks

This chapter concludes this book on IOM which was based on our experience with the IOM service at Hermann Hospital in Houston, Texas, U.S.A., and on the collective experience of other centers. From the very beginning, rather than being exhaustive, we decided to present a general overview of the most typical and effective neurophysiological tests currently in use, the principles on which they are based, the specific surgical procedures that can be applied to, along with some recommendations regarding proper implementation and interpretation of the recordings. Inevitably, however, in doing so we have left out some less frequently used procedures, such as, for instance, monitoring of the pudendal nerve during a prostatectomy. However, this book has provided enough material so that interested readers could easily adapt the techniques presented here to other, more specific cases.

The merits of IOM have been extensively reported in the literature from different institutions worldwide [40, 53, 57, 61]. It is now clear that IOM offers an objective and effective way to assess the functional integrity of the nervous system of patients undergoing orthopedic, neurological, or vascular surgery, and this explains why IOM is gradually becoming part of standard medical practice.

It is our hope, however, that this book has clearly conveyed the message that successful performance of intraopeative monitoring "is *not* simply a matter of bringing another piece of equipment in the operating room" [75]. Rather, it is the application of several complicated neurophysiological procedures, as described in the previous chapters, and the proper interpretation of the results obtained.

There are several factors that contribute to a successful IOM service among which are the following: (1) knowledge about the anatomical and functional characteristics of the structures that generate the signals under study; (2) understanding of the effects of surgical and perisurgical factors on the recordings; (3) properly trained personnel who follow the guidelines set forth by the American Electroencephalographic Society [6]; (4) ability to follow a systematic interventional strategy for recognizing the various types of artifacts and for troubleshooting equipment failures; and finally (5) integration of the monitoring personnel into the surgical and anesthesia teams.

Only then can intraoperative monitoring be used as a safe, very useful, clinically valid, and cost-effective procedure that can improve the outcome of a variety of surgical procedures.

References

[1] Albert, T.J., Balderston, R.A., and Northup, B.E., *Surgical Approaches to the Spine,* W.B. Saunders, Philadelphia, 1997.

[2] An, H.S., Cotler, J.M., and Balderson, R.A., *Complications in Spinal Surgery,* Balderson, R.A. and An, H.S., Eds., W.B. Saunders, Philadelphia, 1991.

[3] Andrews, R.J. and Giffard, R.G., Clinically useful nonanesthetic agents, in *Intraoperative Neuroprotection,* Andrews, R.J., Ed., Williams & Wilkins, Baltimore, 1996.

[4] Andrews, R.J. and Bringas, J.R., A review of brain retraction and recommendations for minimizing intraoperative brain injury, *Neurosurgery,* 33, 1052, 1993.

[5] Andrews, R.J., *Intraoperative Neuroprotection,* Andrews, R.J., Ed., Williams & Wilkins, Baltimore, 1996.

[6] Anon., Guideline eleven: guidelines for intraoperative monitoring of sensory evoked potentials, American Electroencephalographic Society, *J. Clin. Neurophysiol.,* 11, 77, 1994.

[7] Calancie, B., Madsen, P., and Lebwohl, N., Stimulus-evoked EMG monitoring during transpedicular lumbosacral spine instrumentation, *Spine,* 19, 2780, 1993.

[8] Chen, T.C., Maceri, D.R., Levy, M.L., and Giannotta, S.L., Brain stem compression secondary to adipose graft prolapse after translabyrinthine craniotomy: case report, *Neurosurgery,* 35, 521, 1994.

[9] Chiappa, K.H., Evoked potentials in clinical medicine, Chiappa, K.H., Ed., 2nd ed., Raven Press, New York, 1990.

[10] Clements, D.H., Morledge, D.E., Martin, W.H., and Betz, R.R., Evoked and spontaneous electromyography to evaluate lumbosacral pedicle screw placement, *Spine,* 21, 600, 1996.

[11] Cotler, J.M. and Cotler, H.B., *Spinal Fusion, Science and Technique,* Springer-Verlag, New York, 1990.

[12] Craib, A.R. and Most, M., *The EEG Handbook,* Low, M.D., Ed., Beckman Instruments, Vancouver, 1973.

[13] Daspit, C.P., Raudzens, P.A., and Shetter, A.G., Monitoring of intraoperative auditory brain stem responses, *Arch. Otolaryngol. Head Neck Surg.,* 90, 108, 1982.

[14] Delgado, T.E., Bucheit, W.A., Rosenholtz, H.R., and Chrissian, S., Intraoperative monitoring of facial muscle evoked responses obtained by intracranial stimulation of the facial nerve: a more accurate technique for facial nerve dissection, *Neurosurgery,* 4, 418, 1979.

[15] Ebersold, M.J., Harner, S.G., Beatty, C.W., and Harper, C.M. Jr., and Quast, L.M., Current results of the retrosigmoid approach to acoustic neurinoma, *J. Neurosurgery,* 76, 901, 1992.

[16] Engler, G.L., Spielholz, N.J., Bernhard, W.N., Danziger, F., Merkin, H., and Wolff, T., Somatosensory evoked potentials during Harrington instrumentation for scoliosis, *J. Bone Jt. Surg. — Am. Vol.,* 60, 528, 1978.

[17] Esses, S.I., *Textbook of Spinal Disorders,* J.B. Lippincott, Philadelphia, 1995.

[18] Follett, K.A., Intraoperative electrophysiologic spinal cord monitoring, in *Intraoperative Monitoring Techniques in Neurosurgery,* Loftus, C.M. and Traynelis, V.C., Eds., McGraw-Hill, New York, 1994.

[19] Frazier, W.T., Anaesthetic requirements for spinal surgery and effective cord monitoring, in *Handbook of Spinal Cord Monitoring,* Jones, Boyd, Hetreed, and Smith, Eds., Kluwer Academic Publishers, Dordrecht, 1994.

[20] Freye, E., *Cerebral Monitoring in the Operating Room and the Intensive Care Unit,* Kluwer Academic Publishers, Dordrecht, 1990.

[21] Giffard, R.G. and Jaffe, R.A., Anesthetic agents for neuroprotection, in *Intraoperative Neuroprotection,* Andrews, R.J., Ed., Williams & Wilkins, Baltimore, 1996.

[22] Grundy, B.L., Jannetta, P.J., Procopio, P.T., Lina, A., Boston, J.R., and Doyle, E., Intraoperative monitoring of brain-stem auditory evoked potentials, *J. Neurosurg.,* 57, 674, 1982.

[23] Grundy, B.L. and Villani, R.M., *Evoked potentials: intraoperative and ICU monitoring,* Grundy, B.L. and Villani, R.M., Eds., Wien; Springer-Verlag, New York, 1988.

[24] Harner, S.G., Daube, J.R., Ebersold, M.J., and Beatty, C.W., Improved preservation of facial nerve function with use of electrical monitoring during removal of acoustic neuromas, *Mayo Clin. Proc.,* 62, 92, 1987.

[25] Harner, S.G., Beatty, C.W., and Ebersold, M.J., Retrosigmoid removal of acoustic neuroma: experience 1978–1988. *Arch. Otolaryngol. Head Neck Surg.,* 103, 40, 1990.

[26] Jasper, H., Report of committee on methods of clinical exam in EEG, *Electroencephalography and Clinical Neurophysiology,* 10, 370, 1958.

[27] Jewett, D.L. and Williston, J.S., Auditory-evoked far fields averaged from the scalp of humans, *Brain,* 94, 681, 1971.

[28] Kalman, C.J., Been, H.D., and Ongerboer de Visser, B.W., Intraoperative monitoring of spinal cord function, a review, *Acta Orthop. Scand.,* 64, 114, 1993.

[29] Kandel, E.R., Schwartz, J.H., and Jessell, T.M., Eds., *Principles of Neural Science,* 3rd ed., Elsevier, New York, 1991.

[30] Kartush, J.M. and Lundy, L.B., Facial nerve outcome in acoustic neuroma surgery, *Otolaryngol. Clin. N. Am.,* 25, 623, 1992.

[31] Katz, J., *Anesthesiology: A Comprehensive Study Guide,* Katz, J., Ed., McGraw-Hill, New York, 1997.

[32] Keith, R.W., Stambough, J.L., and Awender, S.H., Somatosensory cortical evoked potentials: a review of 100 cases of intraoperative spinal surgery monitoring, *J. Spinal Disorders,* 3, 220, 1990.

[33] Kemink, J.L., LaRouere, M.J., Kileny, P.R., Telian, S.A., and Hoff, J.T., Hearing preservation following suboccipital removal of acoustic neuromas, *Laryngoscope,* 100, 597, 1990.

[34] Kooi, K.A., Spontaneous electrical activity of the normal brain, in *Fundamentals of Electroencephalography,* Kooi, K.A., Tucker, R.P., Marshall, R.E., Eds., 2nd ed., Harper & Row, Hagerstown: Medical Dept., 1978.

[35] Levy, W.J., Gugino, K.K.V., Ghaly, R., Draugn, L., and O'Mahoney, T., Electrophysiological monitoring: Spinal surgery, in *Intraoperative Neuroprotection,* Andrews, R.J., Ed., Williams & Wilkins, Baltimore, 1996.

[36] Loftus, C.M. and Traynelis, V.C., *Intraoperative Monitoring Techniques in Neurosurgery,* Loftus, C.M. and Traynelis, V.C., Eds., McGraw-Hill, New York, 1994.

[37] MacEwen, G.D., Bunnel, W.P., and Stiram, K., Acute neurological complications in the treatment of scoliosis: a report of the Scoliosis Research Society, *J. Bone Joint Surg.,* 57, 404, 1975.

[38] Markand, O.N., Brainstem auditory evoked potentials, *J. Clin. Neurophysiol.,* 11, 319, 1994.

[39] Markand, O.N., Continuous assessment of cerebral function with EEG and somatosensory evoked potential techniques during extracranial vascular reconstruction, in *Intraoperative Monitoring Techniques in Neurosurgery,* Loftus, C.M. and Traynelis, V.C., Eds., McGraw-Hill, New York, 1994.

[40] Matsui, Y., Goh, K., Shiiya, N., Murashita, T., Miyama M., Ohba J., Gohda T., Sakuma M., Yasuda K., and Tanabe T., Clinical application of evoked spinal cord potentials elicited by direct stimulation of the cord during temporary occlusion of the thoracic aorta, *J. Thorac. Cardiovasc. Surg.,* 107, 1519, 1994.

[41] McPherson, R.W., Mahla, M., Johnson, R., and Traystman, R.J., Effects of enflurane, isoflurane, and nitrous oxide on somatosensory evoked potentials during fentanyl anesthesia, *Anesthesiology,* 62, 626, 1985.

[42] Niedermeyer, E. and Lopes da Silva, F., Eds., Neuroanesthesia and neurological monitoring, in *Electroencephalography: Basic Principles, Clinical Applications, and Related Fields,* 3rd ed., Williams Williams, Baltimore, 1993.

[43] McPherson, R.W., General anesthetic considerations in intraoperative monitoring: Effects of anesthetic agents and neuromuscular blockade on evoked potentials, EEG, and cerebral blood flow, in *Intraoperative Monitoring Techniques in Neurosurgery,* Loftus, C.M. and Traynelis, V.C., Eds., McGraw-Hill, New York, 1994.

[44] Møller, A.R., *Evoked Potentials in Intraoperative Monitoring,* Møller, A.R., Ed., Williams & Wilkins, Baltimore, 1988.

[45] Møller, A.R., *Intraoperative Neurophysiologic Monitoring in Neurosurgery*, Schramm, J. and Møller, A.R., Eds., Springer-Verlag, Berlin; New York, 1991.

[46] Møller, A.R., Physiology of the auditory system and recording of auditory evoked potentials, in *Neuromonitoring in Otology and Head and Neck Surgery*, Kartush, J.M. and Bouchard, K.R., Eds., Raven Press, New York, 1992.

[47] Møller, A.R., Intraoperative neurophysiologic monitoring of cranial nerves, in *Neurosurgical Topics Book 13, "Surgery of Cranial Nerves of the Posterior Fossa,"* Barrow, D.L., Ed., American Association of Neurological Surgeons, Park Ridge, IL, 1993.

[48] Møller, A.R., Neurophysiologic monitoring: cranial neurosurgery, in *Intraoperative Neuroprotection*, Andrews, R.J., Ed., Williams & Wilkins, Baltimore, 1996.

[49] Møller, A.R. and Jannetta, P.J., Monitoring facial EMG responses during microvascular decompression operations for hemifacial spasm, *J. Neurosurg.*, 66, 681, 1987.

[50] Nadol, J.B., Jr., Diamond, P.F., and Thornton, A.R., Correlation of hearing loss and radiologic dimensions of vestibular schwannomas (acoustic Neuromas), *Am. J. Otol.*, 17, 312, 1996.

[51] Nash, C.L., Jr., Lorig, R.A., Schatzinger, L.A., and Brown, R.H., Spinal cord monitoring during operative treatment of the spine, *Clin. Orthopaed. Related Res.*, 126, 100, 1977.

[52] North, R.B., Drenger, B., Beattie, C., McPherson, R.W., Parker, S., Reitz B.A., and Williams G.M., Monitoring of spinal cord stimulation evoked potentials during thoracoabdominal aneurysm surgery, *Neurosurgery*, 28, 325, 1991.

[53] Nuwer, M.R., Dawson, E.G., Carlson, L.G., Kanim, L.E., and Sherman, J.E., Somatosensory evoked potential spinal cord monitoring reduces neurologic deficits after scoliosis surgery: results of a large multicenter survey, *Electroencephalog. Clin. Neurophysiol.*, 96, 6, 1995.

[54] Owen, J.H., Evoked potential monitoring during spinal surgery, in *The Textbook of Spinal Surgery*, Bridwell, K.H. and DeWald, RoL., Eds., Lippincott, Philadelphia, 1991.

[55] Owen, J.H., Bridwell, K.H., and Lenke, L.G., Innervation pattern of dorsal roots and their effects on the specificity of dermatomal somatosensory evoked potentials, *Spine*, 18, 748, 1993.

[56] Owen, J.H., Kostuik, J.P., Gornet, M., Petr, M., Skelly, J., Smoes, C., Szymanski, J., Townes J., and Wolfe F., The use of mechanically elicited electromyograms to protect nerve roots during surgery for spinal degeneration, *Spine*, 19, 1704, 1994.

[57] Owen, J.H., Sponseller, P.D., Szymanski, J., and Hurdle, M., Efficacy of multimodality spinal cord monitoring during surgery for neuromuscular scoliosis, *Spine*, 20, 1480, 1995.

[58] Aldo, O., *Perotto Anatomical Guide for the Electromyographer: The Limbs and Trunk*, Charles C. Thomas, Springfield, IL, 1994.

[59] Prior, P., The rationale and utility of neurophysiological investigations in clinical monitoring for brain and spinal cord ischemia during surgery and intensive care, *Comp. Meth. Prog. Biomed.*, 51, 13, 1996.

[60] Renshaw, T.S., Idiopathic scoliosis in children, *Curr. Opinion in Pediatr.*, 5, 407, 1993.

[61] Schepens, M.A., Boezeman, E.H., Hamerlijnck, R.P., ter Beek, H., and Vermeulen, F.E., Somatosensory evoked potentials during exclusion and reperfusion of critical aortic segments in thoracoabdominal aortic aneurysm surgery, *J. Cardiac Surg.*, 9, 692, 1994.

[62] Sekiya, T., Hatayama, T., Iwabuchi, T., and Maeda, S., Intraoperative recordings of evoked extraocular muscle activities to monitor ocular motor nerve function, *Neurosurgery*, 32, 227, 1993.

[63] Shelton, C., Brackmann, D.E., House, W.F., and Hitselberger, W.E., Acoustic tumor surgery: prognostic factors in hearing conversation, *Arch. Otolaryngol. Head Neck Surg.*, 115, 1213, 1989.

[64] Slbin, M.S., Babinski, M., Maroon, J.C., and Jannetta, P.J., Anesthetic management of posterior fossa surgery in the sitting position, *Acta. Anaesthesiol. Scand.*, 20, 117, 1976.

[65] Spehlmann, R., *EEG Primer*, Elsevier Biomedical, Amsterdam, 1981.

[66] Spehlmann, R., *Evoked Potential Primer: Visual, Auditory, and Somatosensory Evoked Potentials in Clinical Diagnosis*, Spehlmann, R., Ed., Butterworth, Boston, 1985.

[67] Staudt, L.A., Nuwer, M.R., and Peacock, W.J., Intraoperative monitoring during selective posterior rhizotomy: technique and patient outcome, *Electroencephal. Clin. Neurophys.*, 97, 296, 1995.

[68] Stephen, J.P., Sullivan, M.R., Hicks, R.G., Burke, D.J., Woodforth, I.J., and Crawford, M.R., Cotrel–Dubousset instrumentation in children using simultaneous motor and somatosensory evoked potential monitoring, *Spine*, 21, 2450, 1996.

[69] Strauss, C., Fahlbusch, R., Nimsky, C., and Cedzich, C., Monitoring visual evoked potentials during para- and suprasellar procedures, in *Intraoperative Monitoring Techniques in Neurosurgery*, Loftus, C.M. and Traynelis, V.C., Eds., McGraw-Hill, New York, 1994.

[70] Tempelhoff, R. and Cheng, M.A., EEG Monitoring, in *Intraoperative Neuroprotection*, Andrews, R.J., Ed., Williams & Wilkins, Baltimore, 1996.

[71] Toleikis, J.R., Carlvin, A.O., Shapiro, D.E., and Schafer, M.F., The use of dermatomal evoked responses during surgical procedures that use intrapedicular fixation of the lumbosacral spine, *Spine*, 18, 2401, 1993.

[72] Tortora, G.J. and Evans, R.L., *Principles of Human Physiology*, 2nd ed., Harper & Row, New York, 1986.

[73] Tyner, F.S., *Fundamentals of EEG Technology*, Tyner, F.S., Knott, J.R., Mayer, W.B., Jr., Tyner, F.S., Eds., Raven Press, New York, 1983.

[74] Watkins, R.G., *The Spine in Sports*, Mosby, St. Louis, MI, 1996.

[75] Yingling, C.D. and Gardi, J.N., Intraoperative monitoring of facial and cochlear nerves during acoustic neuroma surgery, *Otolaryngol. Clin. of North Am.,* 25, 413, 1992.

[76] Young, M.L., Smith, D.S., Murtagh, F., Vasquez, A., and Levitt, J., Comparison of surgical and anesthetic complications in neurosurgical patients experiencing venous air embolism in the sitting position, *Neurosurgery,* 18(2), 157, 1986.

[77] Young, W. and Mollin, D., Intraoperative somatosensory evoked potentials monitoring of spinal surgery, in *Neuromonitoring in Surgery,* Desmedt, J.E., Ed., Elsevier, Amsterdam, 1989.

Further Reading

1. Burke, D. and Hicks, R.G., Surgical monitoring of motor pathways, *J. Clin. Neurophysiol.,* 15, 194, 1998.

2. Cioni, B., Meglio, M., and Rossi, G.F., *Intraoperative motor evoked potentials monitoring in spinal neurosurgery, Arch. Ital. Biol.,* 137, 115, 1999.

3. de Haan, P., Kalkman, C.J., and Jacobs, M.J., Spinal cord monitoring with myogenic motor evoked potentials: early detection of spinal cord ischemia as an integral part of spinal cord protective strategies during thoracoabdominal aneurysm surgery, *Semin. Thorac. Cardiovasc. Surg.,* 10, 19, 1998.

4. Deutsch, H., Arginteanu, M., Manhart, K., Perin, N., Camins, M., Moore, F., Steinberger, A.A., and Weisz, D.J., Somatosensory evoked potential monitoring in anterior thoracic vertebrectomy, *J. Neurosurg.,* 92, 155, 2000.

5. Gharagozloo, F., Neville, R.F., Jr., and Cox, J.L., Spinal cord protection during surgical procedures on the descending thoracic and thoracoabdominal aorta: a critical overview, *Semin. Thorac. Cardiovasc. Surg.,* 10, 73, 1998.

6. Harper, C.M. and Daube, J.R., Facial nerve electromyography and other cranial nerve monitoring, *J. Clin. Neurophysiol.,* 15, 206, 1998.

7. Holland, N.R., Intraoperative electromyography during thoracolumbar spinal surgery, *Spine,* 23, 1915, 1998.

8. Kartush, J.M., Intra-operative monitoring in acoustic neuroma surgery, *Neurol. Res.,* 20, 593, 1998.

9. Nuwer, M.R., Spinal cord monitoring, *Muscle Nerve,* 22, 1620, 1999.

10. Padberg, A.M. and Bridwell, K.H., Spinal cord monitoring: current state of the art, *Orthop. Clin. North Am.,* 30, 407, 1999.

11. Robertazzi, R.R. and Cunningham, J.N., Jr., Monitoring of somatosensory evoked potentials: a primer on the intraoperative detection of spinal cord ischemia during aortic reconstructive surgery, *Semin. Thorac. Cardiovasc. Surg.,* 10, 11, 1998.

12. Rossini, P.M. and Rossi, S. Clinical applications of motor evoked potentials, *Electroencephalogr. Clin. Neurophysiol.,* 106, 180, 1998.

13. Schlake, H.P., Goldbrunner, R., Milewski, C., Siebert, M., Behr, R., Riemann, R., Helms, J., and Roosen, K., Technical developments in intra-operative monitoring for the preservation of cranial motor nerves and hearing in skull base surgery, *Neurol. Res.,* 21, 11, 1999.

14. Slimp, J.C., Intraoperative monitoring of nerve repairs, *Hand. Clin.,* 16(1), 25, 2000.

15. Sloan, T.B., Anesthetic effects on electrophysiologic recordings, *J. Clin. Neurophysiol.,* 5, 217, 1998.

16. Stump, D.A., Jones, T.J., and Rorie, K.D., Neurophysiologic monitoring and outcomes in cardiovascular surgery, *J. Cardiothorac. Vasc. Anesth.,* 13, 600, 1999.

17. Taylor, C.L. and Selman, W.R., Temporary vascular occlusion during cerebral aneurysm surgery, *Neurosurg. Clin. N. Am.,* 9, 673, 1998.

Index